Daily
Aromatherapy

Other books by Joni Keim and Ruah Bull

Aromatherapy & Subtle Energy Techniques: Compassionate Healing with Essential Oils
Aromatherapy Anointing Oils: Spiritual Blessings, Ceremonies, and Affirmations

Daily Aromatherapy

Transforming
the Seasons of Your Life
with Essential Oils

JONI KEIM & RUAH BULL

North Atlantic Books
Berkeley, California

Published by
North Atlantic Books   Cover photo © istockphoto/RalphTV
P.O. Box 12327   Cover design © Gia Giasullo
Berkeley, California 94712   Book design © Ayelet Maida

Printed in the United States of America

Daily Aromatherapy: Transforming the Seasons of Your Life with Essential Oils is sponsored by the Society for the Study of Native Arts and Sciences, a nonprofit educational corporation whose goals are to develop an educational and crosscultural perspective linking various scientific, social, and artistic fields; to nurture a holistic view of arts, sciences, humanities, and healing; and to publish and distribute literature on the relationship of mind, body, and nature.

North Atlantic Books' publications are available through most bookstores. For further information, call 800-337-2665 or visit our website at www.northatlanticbooks.com.

Substantial discounts on bulk quantities are available to corporations, professional associations, and other organizations. For details and discount information, contact our special sales department.

Library of Congress Cataloging-in-Publication Data
Keim, Joni, 1950–
    Daily aromatherapy : transforming the seasons of your life with essentialoils / by Joni Keim and Ruah Bull.
        p. cm.
    Summary: "A gift book, organized by season, that presents 365 daily intention exercises that bring nature's aromas and their positive, transformative qualities into one's life, showing how the action of the essential oils can change your state of mind and help you achieve a sense of well-being in your body, mind, heart, and spirit"—Provided by publisher.
    ISBN 978-1-55643-693-2
    1. Aromatherapy—Calendars. 2. Essences and essential oils—Calendars. 3. Seasons. I. Bull, Ruah, 1951– II. Title.
RM666.A68K38 2008
615'.3219—dc22

                            2007039055

1 2 3 4 5 6 7 8 9 VERSA 15 14 13 12 11 10 09 08

To my children

Travis—my son, the first born, the Gemini, the sun, the ebullient spirit, the wizard.

Annie—my daughter, the second born, the Libra, the moon, the distant star, the high priestess.

–Joni Keim

To Lynn Breedlove, whose living and dying taught me the preciousness of each day, and Becky Green, who continues to show me how to honor the seasons.

–Ruah Bull

Acknowledgments

My gratitude and appreciation to:

Ruah, for her commitment to this book, which completes our trilogy, and for her friendship on this journey of exploration, discovery, hard work, and manifesting our goal.

Gail Atkins, for taking the time, once again, to help us with her valuable editing skills.

Christopher Bolt, long-lost friend, for his photography skills and graciously spending the time with me to get the "right" picture.

–Joni Keim

My gratitude and appreciation to:

Les, for his love that supports me in every season.

My father, who continues to teach me about spirituality.

Jean, Nancy, and Joanna, who have helped me to reconnect to the contemplative dimension of Christianity.

Joni, as always, my friend and colleague and co-writer, who keeps me organized, focused, and edited—all the while having great fun.

–Ruah Bull

Contents

❧ Autumn ☙

❧ Winter ❧

Note: Aromatherapy is a wholistic modality, affecting the body, mind, emotions, and spirit. The focus of this book is on the mental, emotional, and spiritual effects of essential oils. The physical effects, such as which oils to use for colds and flu or muscle strain, are not included. We do believe, however, that physical health is affected positively by mental, emotional, and spiritual well-being.

The information in this book is intended to assist you in achieving positive changes in your life and creating a sense of well-being. It is in no way intended to replace professional medical or psychological care.

Foreword

Time moves along. We feel its passage as we gaze back at yesterday, last week, last year. The cycles and seasons ahead of us, our very future days, are in our minds and hearts already. The seasons mark our days and bring to life our inner clock. We feel our spirit's journey, and we faintly hear our soul's timepiece—moving us toward our destiny.

But how do we experience time—its pace, its movement, its passage, and its flow? What is our relationship to it? Does that relationship reside in stress and discord? Or can we experience time in a healthful way—a way that will wake us to a sense of unity, peace, and harmony in our life? Can we experience it with a sense of connectedness to nature—the cycles, the diversity, and the wisdom? Can we be present in every moment? Perhaps we can—this day, this month, this very season.

The course of this book brings us to a new relationship with *our time.* It awakens our senses as we journey through the seasons—the seasons of the year and the seasons of our souls. We are embraced by their power, their beauty, and their wisdom—as they flow in, around, and through us. The authors have chosen natural plant extracts, known as essential oils, to guide and accompany us. We benefit from their guidance, we enjoy their companionship, and we long for their affirmations that sing out to us. They are reminders that we are part of a larger creation, held close in connection to the passing of the seasons and to time without end.

This creative and inspired book offers us profound experiences that gently penetrate to the roots and wings of our being. It is written with insight, wisdom, generosity, wit, and reverence. The innovative, guided exercises are a powerful selection of self-healing journeys that will surely transport us to a full, rich, and deep understanding of the gentle way that healing can occur—for ourselves, our families, our loved ones, and our world. The inspirational tone—awakening us to the preparation, calling, and accepting of the seasons—is ringing the right chimes at the right time. We are being given a unique opportunity and approach to healing that promises many good blessings.

Time moves along. We feel its passage as we gaze back at yesterday, last week, last year. The cycles and seasons ahead of us, our very future days, are in our minds and hearts already. The seasons mark our days and bring to life our inner clock. Move forward now in the pages of this book toward your destiny, and may you gather the blessings and wisdom of its teachings.

Becky Ann Green, PhD
Director, Twin Lakes College, Santa Cruz
mid-Winter 2007

·

Introduction

*D*aily Aromatherapy: Transforming the Seasons of Your
Life with Essential Oils brings nature's aromas and
their positive-transformation abilities into your life on a daily
basis. *Transforming,* as it is used in this book, means *changing your state of mind* or *shifting your consciousness.* Combined with your *intention—what you passionately want to
achieve*—the exercises in this book can assist you in every
aspect of your life—from feeling secure in the world to
strengthening your spirituality. They can help you achieve a
sense of wholeness and well-being. They can help you heal.

In 2002, at an aromatherapy conference in San Francisco,
Jeffrey Yuen, a master of classical Chinese medicine, spoke
on "Chinese Medical Aromatherapy." His lecture was profound and inspiring. He explained that essential oils are used
in Traditional Chinese Medicine (TCM) in a variety of ways
and that one of the key ways was for *transformation.* He said
unequivocally that "one cannot use essential oils *without*
being transformed." The oils work well because they "connect with the essence of an individual by activating the
senses." Continuing, he said that *true healing* is about connection and transformation, and using essential oils is an invitation to heal. The exercises in *Daily Aromatherapy* embrace
these concepts.

Using aromas to shift your consciousness is not new. In fact, they have been used through the ages by many cultures to assist in a variety of transformation techniques such as meditation, affirmation, visualization, spirit journeys, and prayer. Incense and fragrant herbs are still used in Christian churches and Buddhist temples, and by Tibetans and Native Americans.

When we use essential oils for transformation, we rely on their aromas to create a psychological response following an intention. As Yuen explained, "Your intention creates your experience." When aromas are inhaled through the nose, odor molecules are received by the olfactory epithelium (at the top of the nose, inside), which transmits nerve impulses to the limbic brain. Here, they produce and evoke emotional feelings, emotional states, and physical responses. These are determined by the experience associated with that oil and, to some degree, by the oil's biochemical constituents. When aromas are used with a positive, transformational intent, a connection is made and stored in this area of the brain. The intent can be reexperienced when the aroma is inhaled again, and the more often the aroma is used with the intent, the stronger the connection.

When assigning an association or theme to a particular essential oil for transformation, we base it on the oil's subtle energy properties that affect the subtle anatomy (the energy centers and energy fields) associated with the human body. The subtle energy properties gently coax erratic cellular vibration into a harmonious or intended vibration. Subtle energy properties are determined by taking into consideration the long-term, traditional uses of both the essential oil and herb of the plant, the physical and psychological effects of the oil, the color of the oil, the gesture and signature of the plant itself (its appearance and characteristics), and personal experience.

As we explore the subtle properties of the essential oils, the format of *Daily Aromatherapy* follows the seasons of the year as they correlate to the symbolic seasons of the evolving human soul. Spring is the season of optimism and new beginnings. It is the time to clear away the old and begin anew. It represents the hopeful, childhood years. Summer is the season of activity and manifesting goals and desires. It represents the dynamic young-adult years. Autumn is the season to reflect on life, to accept, to forgive, and to heal. It represents the insightful, mid-life years. Winter is the season to rest, restore, and rejuvenate, and to prioritize and focus on what is most dear. Winter represents the wise and spiritual senior years.

Daily Aromatherapy begins with the Spring months, followed by those of Summer, Autumn, and Winter. Each month of the year profiles and explores four different essential oils—one per week. Every essential oil is identified by its common name, its Latin name, and its best transformational use. The part of the plant from which the oil is extracted, such as the leaf, seed, flower, or wood, is noted. Most importantly, the essential oil's psychological (mental, emotional) and subtle (energetic) properties are listed. Designated in the subtle properties are the animals and archangels that align with particular essential oils; these will be helpful for those who resonate with the animal kingdom and the angelic realm.

You will experience and come to know each of the forty-eight essential oils very well by doing seven different intention exercises, one per day for a week: an affirmation, emotional self-discovery questions, a ceremony, a blessing, an activity, a visualization, and a prayer.

1. The affirmation exercise uses a positively worded statement to help mobilize your inner resources to make helpful changes in your life. It describes what you want in the present moment, as if it is already a reality.

2. The emotional self-discovery exercise uses self-reflection questions that you contemplate and answer. They are designed to help you explore and understand your emotions.

3. There are four different types of ceremony exercises per month: clearing, attracting, integrating, and manifesting. The *clearing* ceremony helps you to clear away and release obstacles that prevent you from reaching your desired goal. The *attracting* ceremony helps you create an internal and external experience that draws your desired goal to you. The *integrating* ceremony helps you to fully embody your intentions to reach your desired goal. The

manifesting ceremony helps complete the intention process and brings your desired goal into reality.

4. The blessing exercise is a statement that honors your intention as holy, asking that it be protected and enhanced.

5. The activity exercise is your body in motion or action, in some specific way, to help bring your desired goal to reality.

6. The visualization exercise uses your imagination to create positive, internal pictures, helping you to create what you want in your life and to make constructive changes.

7. The prayer exercise is a statement addressed to the Divine.

At the end of each month, the number of remaining days varies, so the exercises and essential oils also vary. Four additional, new essential oils are profiled in these end-of-the-month days, one per season, making a total of fifty-two essential oils explored in the book. Besides the new essential oil exercise, you may be guided to *write* an affirmation, celebrate the season, meditate, honor your accomplishments, or make a special essential oil blend. When making a blend, keep in mind that the number of drops chosen for each essential oil is intended to create an aesthetically pleasing aroma. It does not mean that there will be more of one quality, such as "forgiveness," and less of another, such as "protection," in the blend. In subtle aromatherapy, it is the energy of the essential oil, not the quantity, that is important.

In all of the intention exercises for the year, you will be asked to smell the aroma of an essential oil—one drop on a tissue. In some cases, you will be asked to smell the aroma more than once. This is a transformational experience, as described above, but for the experience to be the best it can be, it requires that you are able to receive. Many people involved with essential oils are givers, nurturers, and helpers who know well how to give of themselves for others. However, many do not know how to receive well. *Receiving* is the energetic balance of *giving.* If you cannot fully receive, you cannot fully give. In addition, we believe that in order to be "available" for intuitive information and spiritual guidance, you need to be able to receive. The exercises in this book are an excellent opportunity for you to practice, develop, and deepen your capacity to receive.

Upon completion of *Daily Aromatherapy,* we have completed our trilogy, which began with *Aromatherapy & Subtle Energy Techniques* (2000) and *Aromatherapy Anointing Oils* (2001). We have worked with aromatherapy for more than twenty years and have been deeply moved by the generous spirit of essential oils and their profound ability to improve our lives. They have been our healers, teachers, and friends. May they be a blessing to you, in the days and seasons of your life, as they have been to us.

How to Use This Book

*D*aily Aromatherapy can be used in a variety of ways, and we invite you to explore them all. You may choose to use it on a daily, weekly, monthly, or seasonal basis or just for special occasions. You may simply want to get to know specific essential oils very well and focus on just those, or work on transforming one aspect of your life. In the process, you may discover or create new ways to use the oils that suit your individual needs. In whatever way you choose to use this book, please enjoy and experience the blessings of essential oils as they guide you through the seasons of your life.

~ The Essential Oils ~

Following is a list of the essential oils used in *Daily Aromatherapy.* There are a total of fifty-two, and both their common and botanical names are given. You do not need to have all these oils to enjoy or use this book, but you will need at least one to get started. (See "Specific Choice," below.) They appear here in alphabetical order, rather than the order of their use in the book. Essential oils are available at natural food stores, at specialty shops, and direct from essential oil companies.

Some essential oil specialists feel that your preference for an aroma can be an accurate guide for what you need—that you will be drawn to the aroma of an essential oil that will be of benefit to you. Conversely, you will be repelled by an aroma that will not benefit you. Indeed, if you do not like the aroma of a particular oil, it will likely not create a positive experience if you use it. Though your psyche could probably be trained to accept the oil, these exercises are intended to be enjoyable, so if you do not care for the aroma of an oil, please see Appendix II: Alternate and Additional Best Essential Oils and choose another, appropriate one.

Basil *(Ocimum basilicum)*
Bay Laurel *(Laurus nobilis)*
Bay St. Thomas *(Pimenta racemosa)*
Benzoin *(Styrax benzoin)*
Bergamot *(Citrus bergamia)*
Cardamom *(Elettaria cardamomum)*
Cedarwood *(Cedrus atlantica)*
Champaca *(Michelia champaca)*
Cinnamon *(Cinnamomum verum)*
Clary Sage *(Salvia sclarea)*
Clove *(Eugenia caryophyllata)*
Coriander *(Coriandrum sativum)*
Cypress *(Cupressus sempervirens)*
Elemi *(Canarium luzonicum)*
Eucalyptus *(Eucalyptus globulus)*
Fennel *(Foeniculum vulgare dulce)*
Fir *(Abies balsamea)*
Frankincense *(Boswellia carterii)*
Geranium *(Pelargonium graveolens)*

German Chamomile *(Matricaria chamomilla)*
Ginger *(Zingiber officinale)*
Grapefruit *(Citrus paradisi)*
Immortelle *(Helichrysum italicum)*
Jasmine *(Jasminum officinale)*
Juniper Berry *(Juniperus communis)*
Lavender *(Lavandula vera/officinalis)*
Lemon *(Citrus limonum)*
Lemongrass *(Cymbopogon citratus)*
Mandarin *(Citrus reticulata var. mandarin)*
Marjoram *(Origanum majorana)*
Mimosa *(Acacia dealbata)*
Myrrh *(Commiphora myrrha)*
Neroli *(Citrus aurantium)*
Nutmeg *(Myristica fragrans)*
Oakmoss *(Evernia prunastri)*
Orange *(Citrus sinensis)*
Palmarosa *(Cymbopogon martini)*
Peppermint *(Mentha piperita)*
Petitgrain *(Citrus aurantium var. amara)*
Pine *(Pinus sylvestris)*
Roman Chamomile *(Anthemis nobilis)*
Rose *(Rosa damascena)*
Rosemary *(Rosmarinus officinalis)*
Rosewood *(Aniba rosaeodora)*
Sandalwood *(Santalum album)*
Spikenard *(Nardostachys jatamansi)*
Spruce *(Picea mariana)*
Tea Tree *(Melaleuca alternifolia)*
Thyme *(Thymus vulgaris)*
Vanilla *(Vanilla planifolia)*
Vetiver *(Vetiveria zizanioides)*
Ylang Ylang *(Cananga odorata)*

❧ Nine Different Ways ❧ to Use this Book

Daily

You will need all fifty-two essential oils.

As a part of your daily routine, follow the days of the calendar year. For example, if it is January 27, do the exercise for that day.

Weekly

You will need forty-eight essential oils—all of them except Mimosa, Champaca, Immortelle, and German Chamomile. (These are the "new" essential oils that are used in the end-of-the-month exercises.)

Do the exercise on days one, eight, fifteen, and twenty-two of every month. These dates have the affirmations of four different essential oils.

Monthly

You will need twelve essential oils. Choose one essential oil per month and do one or more of the exercises for that essential oil. Following are suggestions for each month.

Spring
    ❧ For March, do one or more of the exercises for Lemongrass.

- For April, do one or more of the exercises for Orange.
- For May, do one or more of the exercises for Geranium.

Summer

- For June, do one or more of the exercises for Rosemary.
- For July, do one or more of the exercises for Thyme.
- For August, do one or more of the exercises for Ginger.

Autumn

- For September, do one or more of the exercises for Spruce.
- For October, do one or more of the exercises for Lavender.
- For November, do one or more of the exercises for Rose.

Winter

- For December, do one or more of the exercises for Benzoin.
- For January, do one or more of the exercises for Neroli.
- For February, do one or more of the exercises for Frankincense.

To Experience the Essence of a Season

You will need four essential oils, as listed below.

- ⤚ For Spring, do one or more of the exercises for Geranium.
- ⤚ For Summer, do one or more of the exercises for Thyme.
- ⤚ For Autumn, do one or more of the exercises for Lavender.
- ⤚ For Winter, do one or more of the exercises for Frankincense.

Special Day(s)

You will need one or more essential oils, depending on which days you choose to celebrate.

Find the date that is special for you. It may be your birthday or a special anniversary. Collect the essential oil(s) you will need, and do the exercise for that day.

Random Day(s)

You will need to have the essential oil(s) for the random day(s) you select.

Do the exercise(s) on any day(s) of the year, whichever one(s) you want, whenever you want.

Soul Season

Your soul season is not the same as the actual calendar season. Your soul season represents where you are in your life at this time. This could be your literal age or it could be your emotional age. As you read the descriptions below, choose one that is your literal time of life or one that resonates with you emotionally.

You will need the three essential oils that are indicated for the three months in the chosen season, as recommended in "Monthly" above, or you will need the twelve essential oils, one per week, in your chosen season.

1. Spring is the season of the soul that signals optimism and hope. It is a time to clear away and release what no longer serves you—physically, mentally, emotionally, and spiritually—so that you can experience rebirth, inspiration, and renewed creativity. It is a time for new beginnings, new experiences, new relationships, and new perspectives on existing relationships. Spring is the season that represents the feminine, and also the childhood stage of your life.

2. Summer is the season of the soul that signals manifestation and full expression—the foundation for which is mental clarity, concentration, and focus. Your body, mind, heart, and spirit are energized and motivated, moving your thoughts

into action. Fortitude, courage, and confidence help to bring your heart and soul's desire to fruition. Summer is the season that symbolizes the masculine and represents the young-adult stage of your life.

3. Autumn is the season of the soul that signals a time to reflect on your life and assess the health and well-being of your body, mind, heart, and spirit. It is a time for insights and using good judgment regarding your relationships, how you take care of yourself, how you spend your time, and what you have accomplished. Forgiving and accepting your shortcomings, as well as the shortcomings of others, help you pave the way to a peaceful heart. It is also a time to acknowledge and be grateful for the many blessings in your life, and to be generous of spirit. In all of this, healing takes place. Autumn represents the mid-life stage of your life.

4. Winter is the season of the soul that signals rest. It is a time to feel comfortable, safe, and secure—in body, mind, heart, and spirit. A sense of being *home* embraces you. There is an awareness of wholeness, satisfaction, and abundance. It is a time of peace and trust, and in that, there is restoration and rejuvenation. It is a time when increasing wisdom can lead the way to contemplative spirituality. Winter is the season that represents the senior stage of your life.

As an Oracle

You will need all the essential oils.

The word *oracle* is derived from the Latin verb *orare,* which means "to speak." An oracle, as we use it here, is a source of wise counsel that can tell you what you need to know, when you need to know it. Often, it is something you already know, consciously or subconsciously, but need to be reminded of.

Hold the book in your hands, close your eyes, and take three slow, relaxed, deep breaths. Ask that you be directed to the intention exercise that would most benefit you on this day. Keeping your eyes closed, thumb through the pages of the book until you are guided to stop. Open your eyes. This is the exercise to do, using the assigned essential oil.

Specific Choice

You will need one essential oil. This may be your favorite essential oil or an oil that you just want to get to know better.

In this book, find the essential oil you have chosen, and do the exercises, one per day, for seven days.

Notes: For some of the exercises, it may be helpful to have a friend read them to you slowly as you do them, especially the visualizations. You can also tape them and then play them back.

Be aware that when you are using essential oils, there are safety guidelines to follow. See Appendix VII for general aromatherapy safety recommendations. Essential oils are highly concentrated, and aromatherapy protocol states that they be diluted before use on the skin. However, in this book, the essential oils do not come in contact with your skin; therefore, they are used without being diluted. Their aromas are experienced by smelling one drop from a tissue.

"Take three slow, relaxed, deep breaths" is repeated throughout the book. Deep breathing is taught in many ways. For this book, we suggest the following: Staying relaxed, inhale slowly through your nose to the count of three. Feel your breath deeply fill your abdomen, stomach, and chest. Pause and hold your breath to the count of three. Then, exhale slowly through your nose to the count of three. Feel your breath emptying out of your abdomen, stomach, and chest. Pause to the count of three and then repeat. Do this in a very relaxed, easy manner. Do not force or strain your breathing.

In this book, there are various exercises in which we ask you to take notes. You may want to keep a special notebook just for this purpose, to maintain an account of your responses so you are able to review them later, if needed. It can be particularly interesting in review to note the difference in your responses to an oil at one point in time compared to a later point in time.

Spring

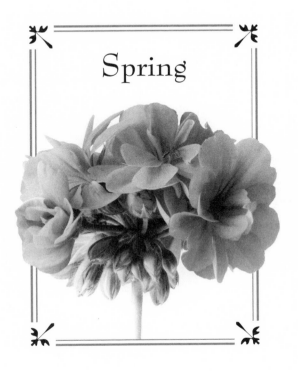

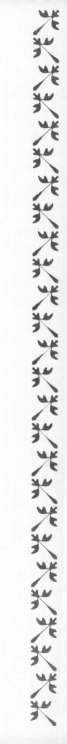

The Spring Months
March, April, May

Spring is the season of the soul that signals optimism and hope. It is a time to clear away and release what no longer serves you—physically, mentally, emotionally, and spiritually—so that you can experience rebirth, inspiration, and renewed creativity. It is a time for new beginnings, new experiences, new relationships, and new perspectives on existing relationships. Spring is the season that represents the feminine, and also the childhood stage of your life.

❧ March ❧

March is the first Spring month—a time for clearing, cleansing, and releasing, so that you can move forward, unburdened, toward your hopes and dreams. The essential oils for this month are Lemongrass to clear and cleanse, Bay St. Thomas for releasing fear, Grapefruit for releasing negative emotions, and Juniper Berry for protecting against negativity.

Lemongrass

Best essential oil to clear and cleanse.

*We must be willing to get rid
of the life we've planned, so as to have
the life that is waiting for us.*
–Joseph Campbell

LATIN NAME: *Cymbopogon citratus*

EXTRACTED FROM: Leaves

PSYCHOLOGICAL PROPERTIES: Uplifts yet calms. Revitalizes and refreshes. Eases minor depression. Relieves irritability and stress. Relieves mental fatigue and jet lag.

SUBTLE PROPERTIES: Clears and cleanses. Uplifts. Promotes optimism and dispels negative energy. Releases regrets and emotional blockages. Associated with the vulture in the animal kingdom.

MARCH 1
Aromatic affirmation with Lemongrass

Sit quietly. Close your eyes. Take three slow, relaxed, deep breaths. Open your eyes. Put a drop of Lemongrass on a tissue and inhale the aroma through your nose. Pause and inhale again.

Say out loud or internally the following affirmation: "It is safe for me now to clear away and gently release what no longer serves me."

Lemongrass helps you to clear away and release outmoded and unnecessary ways of thinking.

MARCH 2
Aromatic emotional self-discovery with Lemongrass

Sit quietly. Close your eyes. Take three slow, relaxed, deep breaths. Open your eyes. Put a drop of Lemongrass on a tissue and inhale the aroma through your nose. Pause and inhale again. Ask yourself the following questions and jot down your answers on a piece of paper.

- What does "clear and cleanse" mean to me?
- Are there emotional reactions to past situations that I am able to clear and cleanse? If so, what are they?
- Are there emotional reactions to past situations that I am unable to clear and cleanse? If so, what are they and why am I still holding onto them?
- What emotions would I like to be able to clear and cleanse?
- How does clearing and cleansing away unwanted emotional blocks benefit me?

Inhale the aroma of Lemongrass again and intend that you are breathing in the ability to clear, cleanse, and release. Review your answers to the above questions. Reflect and jot down any additional notes.

Lemongrass helps you to clear away and release feelings and emotional blockages that are not beneficial for you.

MARCH 3
Aromatic clearing ceremony with Lemongrass

While standing comfortably with your feet slightly apart, close your eyes. Take three slow, relaxed, deep breaths. Open your eyes. Put a drop of Lemongrass on a tissue and inhale the aroma through your nose. Pause and inhale again. With your dominant hand, make three counterclockwise circles (up on the left, down on the right) in front of your forehead, then your heart, and lastly, your stomach area (without touching). Then, raise your hand in front of your mouth and blow forcefully across your palm with the intention that you are releasing all negative energy and negative thoughts. Inhale the aroma again. Feel cleansed of negativity.

Lemongrass helps you to clear away negativity, while releasing emotional blockages.

MARCH 4
Aromatic blessing with Lemongrass

Sit quietly. Close your eyes. Take three slow, relaxed, deep breaths. Open your eyes. Put a drop of Lemongrass on a tissue and inhale the aroma through your nose. Pause and inhale again. Place your right hand over your heart, and say out loud or internally: "Bless my heart and free me of the wounds that keep me from loving unconditionally."

Lemongrass helps you to release thoughts and emotions that interfere with your ability to love.

Aromatic activity with Lemongrass

Sit quietly. Close your eyes. Take three slow, relaxed, deep breaths. Think of one incident, thought, or feeling that needs to be spoken out loud in order to be released. This may be something recent or from the distant past. It could be correcting a lie, righting a wrong, or telling someone you care about them. Hold it in your mind. Open your eyes. Put a drop of Lemongrass on a tissue and inhale the aroma through your nose. Pause and inhale again. Stand up and speak out loud, openly and freely, what it is you want and need to say. You may say it in few words or in many. When you are finished, sense how you are feeling. Describe your feelings out loud.

Lemongrass helps you to release what you want and need to release.

MARCH 6
Aromatic visualization with Lemongrass

Sit quietly. Close your eyes. Take three slow, relaxed, deep breaths. Open your eyes. Put a drop of Lemongrass on a tissue and inhale the aroma through your nose. Pause and inhale again. Close your eyes again. Visualize a beautiful garden. Imagine weeding and cleaning out this garden. Do any trees or bushes need pruning to remove old, dry twigs and leaves? Are there any plants that need to be removed entirely? As you tend to this garden, know that you are making positive changes in yourself—clearing away perceptions and emotions that are no longer needed, allowing for new ideas and growth. Stand back and look at this garden, cleaned and cleared.

Lemongrass helps you to clear away mental and emotional blocks so that you are ready for new personal growth.

MARCH 7
Aromatic prayer with Lemongrass

Sit quietly. Close your eyes. Take three slow, relaxed, deep breaths. Open your eyes. Put a drop of Lemongrass on a tissue and inhale the aroma through your nose. Pause and inhale again. Pray out loud or internally: "Dear God, help me to clear my body, mind, heart, and spirit of all that prevents me from being a conscious and loving instrument in Your name. Help me to keep my consciousness and soul clear so that I may serve only You. Amen."

Lemongrass helps you to surrender and release emotions and thoughts that interfere with your spiritual growth.

Bay St. Thomas

Best essential oil for releasing fear.

> *To conquer fear is*
> *the beginning of wisdom.*
> –Bertrand Russell

LATIN NAME: *Pimenta racemosa*

EXTRACTED FROM: Leaves

PSYCHOLOGICAL PROPERTIES: Promotes mental clarity and
improves concentration. Uplifts. Relieves stress and
anxiety.

SUBTLE PROPERTIES: Clears and cleanses away unwanted
thought patterns and emotional blocks, especially fear.
Associated with the hawk in the animal kingdom.

MARCH 8
Aromatic affirmation with Bay St. Thomas

Sit quietly. Close your eyes. Take three slow, relaxed, deep
breaths. Open your eyes. Put a drop of Bay St. Thomas on
a tissue and inhale the aroma through your nose. Pause and
inhale again.

Say out loud or internally the following affirmation: "I
release all unnecessary fears. I move forward in my life without the fear that hinders."

Bay St. Thomas helps you to release unnecessary fears and
experience the freedom that this brings.

Aromatic emotional self-discovery with Bay St. Thomas

Sit quietly. Close your eyes. Take three slow, relaxed, deep breaths. Open your eyes. Put a drop of Bay St. Thomas on a tissue and inhale the aroma through your nose. Pause and inhale again. Ask yourself the following questions and jot down your answers and reflections on a piece of paper.

- How do I experience fear?
- What fears do I carry from the past that are unnecessary now?
- What beliefs and experiences contribute to my fears?
- How do these fears affect my health? My relationships? My work?
- How will my life be different without these fears?
- How does being free of inappropriate fear benefit me?

Inhale the aroma of Bay St. Thomas again. As you exhale through your mouth, release those fears that you have decided are now unnecessary.

Bay St. Thomas helps you to release fears that are no longer necessary—fears you may have developed from past experiences or that have been learned from others.

MARCH 10
Aromatic attracting ceremony with Bay St. Thomas

Sit quietly. Close your eyes. Take three slow, relaxed, deep breaths. Open your eyes. Put a drop of Bay St. Thomas on a tissue and inhale the aroma through your nose. Pause and inhale again. Light a candle. As you look at the candle, experience its radiant light dispelling the unnecessary fear that dwells in your body, mind, heart, and spirit. Experience the sensation of this freedom in every part of your being. Inhale Bay St. Thomas once again and feel that you are free of the fear that no longer serves you.

Bay St. Thomas helps you to experience the sense of freedom that being free of unnecessary fear can bring.

MARCH 11
Aromatic blessing with Bay St. Thomas

Sit quietly. Close your eyes. Take three slow, relaxed, deep breaths. Open your eyes. Put a drop of Bay St. Thomas on a tissue and inhale the aroma through your nose. Pause and inhale again.

Say out loud or internally: "Bless and strengthen my body so that I can choose trust over fear. Bless and strengthen my mind so that I can choose wisdom over fear. Bless and strengthen my heart so that I can choose love over fear. Bless and strengthen my spirit so that I can choose the Divine over fear."

Bay St. Thomas helps you to let go of old fears that no longer serve a purpose.

Aromatic activity with Bay St. Thomas

Sit quietly. Close your eyes. Take three slow, relaxed, deep breaths. Remember a time when you were afraid to "speak up" about an issue that was important to you. This might be something from your childhood, or something that happened recently in a relationship or at work. Open your eyes. Put a drop of Bay St. Thomas on a tissue and inhale the aroma through your nose. Pause and inhale again. Imagine yourself back in that situation and allow yourself to say out loud everything you wish you had said. Say it as many times as you need to, and in all the ways that you need to. Be sure that you have said all that needs to be said.

Bay St. Thomas helps you to speak courageously about difficult topics.

Aromatic visualization with Bay St. Thomas

Sit quietly. Close your eyes. Take three slow, relaxed, deep breaths. Open your eyes. Put a drop of Bay St. Thomas on a tissue and inhale the aroma through your nose. Pause and inhale again.

Close your eyes again. Visualize a beautiful garden. In the west corner of this garden, find a well of clear, cool, cleansing water. Reach into it. Cup your hands and drink the fresh, healing water. Sense it washing away unnecessary and unwanted fears from the past, both distant and recent. Enjoy this clear state of being. Now, dip your hands in the clear water and drink again. Feel replenished in any part of you that has been depleted by these fears. Know that this sense of replenishment will stay with you for as long as you need.

Bay St. Thomas helps you to clean and clear away unwanted thought patterns and fears that are no longer necessary, allowing you to be nourished and energized.

MARCH 14
Aromatic prayer with Bay St. Thomas

Sit quietly. Close your eyes. Take three slow, relaxed, deep breaths. Open your eyes. Put a drop of Bay St. Thomas on a tissue and inhale the aroma through your nose. Pause and inhale again.

Pray out loud or internally: "Great Spirit, teach me to let go of all fears that separate me from You. Help me to grow daily in courage and in service to You. Amen."

Bay St. Thomas helps you to let go of the fears that separate you from your highest good and from the Divine.

Grapefruit

Best essential oil for releasing negative emotions.

> *Where there is hatred let me sow love;*
> *where there is injury, pardon;*
> *where there is doubt, faith;*
> *where there is despair, hope;*
> *where there is darkness, light;*
> *where there is sadness, joy.*
> –St. Francis of Assisi

LATIN NAME: *Citrus paradisi*

EXTRACTED FROM: Rind

PSYCHOLOGICAL PROPERTIES: Refreshes and uplifts. Relieves
minor depression and mental exhaustion.

SUBTLE PROPERTIES: Releases negative emotions, such as
anger, jealousy, blame, and hatred. Helps dissolve the
energy blocks caused by negative emotions. Clears and
cleanses. Associated with the woodpecker in the animal
kingdom.

MARCH 15
Aromatic affirmation with Grapefruit

Sit quietly. Close your eyes. Take three slow, relaxed, deep
breaths. Open your eyes. Put a drop of Grapefruit on a tissue and inhale the aroma through your nose. Pause and
inhale again. Say out loud or internally the following affirmation: "I release all the conscious and unconscious negativity that prevents me from being a loving human being."

Grapefruit helps you to release negative emotions such as anger, blame, and jealousy.

MARCH 16
Aromatic emotional self-discovery with Grapefruit

Sit quietly. Close your eyes. Take three slow, relaxed, deep breaths. Open your eyes. Put a drop of Grapefruit on a tissue and inhale the aroma through your nose. Pause and inhale again. Ask yourself the following questions and jot down your answers and reflections on a piece of paper.

- What negative emotions am I currently experiencing in my life (for example, anger, jealousy, guilt, resentment)?
- What triggers these emotions for me?
- How do these emotions affect my body, mind, heart, and spirit?
- How will I benefit from releasing these emotions?

Inhale the aroma of Grapefruit again. Choose the most important negative emotion for you to release now. As you exhale through your mouth, let that emotion go and feel what it is like to be free of it.

Grapefruit helps you to release the emotional negativity that burdens you.

Aromatic integrating ceremony with Grapefruit

Sit quietly. Close your eyes. Take three slow, relaxed, deep breaths. Open your eyes. Put a drop of Grapefruit on a tissue and inhale the aroma through your nose. Pause and inhale again. Choose a negative emotion that no longer serves you and that you would like to clear away and release, such as jealousy, anger, blame, or envy. Pour some water into a glass. Hold the glass of water with both hands and intend that it is imbued with light and a positive emotion of your choosing, such as love, forgiveness, or hope. As you drink the water, think: "I release the negative emotion of _____. I am filled with light and the positive emotion of _____ that serves my highest good." When you have finished drinking, experience the spaciousness and freedom created when a negative emotion is released and the sense of well-being created when you integrate a positive emotion.

Grapefruit helps you to clear away and release negative emotions, providing the space for positive emotions.

Aromatic blessing with Grapefruit

Sit quietly. Close your eyes. Take three slow, relaxed, deep breaths. Open your eyes. Put a drop of Grapefruit on a tissue and inhale the aroma through your nose. Pause and inhale again. Think of a person toward whom you have felt negative emotions, such as anger, jealousy, or envy. Say out loud or internally: "Bless [name of person]. May [he/she] be at peace." Inhale the aroma of Grapefruit again. Think of a negative emotion you have toward yourself. Say out loud or internally: "May I be blessed and be at peace."

Grapefruit helps you to release negative emotions that prevent you from being at peace.

MARCH 19
Aromatic activity with Grapefruit

Put 5 drops of Grapefruit around the outer rim of your shower. Turn the shower on and step in. Take three slow, relaxed, deep breaths. Imagine the steam and the Grapefruit enveloping you, helping you identify and then release outdated, unwanted, and unnecessary negative feelings. As you watch the water running down the drain, experience those feelings running down the drain as well. Take three more refreshing breaths and feel the increased energy and sense of freedom you now have. As you dry off after the shower, look forward to experiencing a more positive day.

Grapefruit helps to release the denseness and constriction caused by negative emotions, helping you to experience more energy and a renewed sense of freedom.

MARCH 20
Aromatic visualization with Grapefruit

Sit quietly. Close your eyes. Take three slow, relaxed, deep breaths. Open your eyes. Put a drop of Grapefruit on a tissue and inhale the aroma through your nose. Pause and inhale again. Close your eyes. Visualize a lovely garden. As you look around to enjoy its beauty, a delightful, fresh breeze carries the scent of Grapefruit to you—bright and clear. As you feel, hear, and smell this breeze, sense how the garden itself, and the air in the garden, is being cleansed and refreshed. Notice how the breeze picks up the dried leaves and bits of yard waste and takes them away. Experience this for yourself. Allow the breeze to carry away negative thoughts and emotions. Let the breeze gently waft around and past you for as long as you like. Feel cleansed and refreshed.

Grapefruit helps to release negative patterns of thoughts and beliefs, and refreshes your mind.

MARCH 21
Aromatic prayer with Grapefruit

Sit quietly. Close your eyes. Take three slow, relaxed, deep breaths. Open your eyes. Put a drop of Grapefruit on a tissue and inhale the aroma through your nose. Pause and inhale again. Pray out loud or internally: "Dear God, thank You for helping me to release the negative emotions that harm my body, mind, heart, and spirit. Thank You for all the ways in which You refresh my spirit. Amen."

Grapefruit helps to cleanse away and release negative emotions that prevent you from being at peace and in harmony with the Divine.

Juniper Berry

Best essential oil for protecting against negativity.

> *The happiness of your life depends*
> *upon the quality of your thoughts,*
> *therefore guard accordingly; and take*
> *care that you entertain no notions*
> *unsuitable to virtue ...*
> –Marcus Aurelius Antoninus

LATIN NAME: *Juniperus communis*

EXTRACTED FROM: Berries

PSYCHOLOGICAL PROPERTIES: Emotionally strengthens and uplifts. Relieves anxiety, stress, and nervous tension.

SUBTLE PROPERTIES: Protects against negativity and negative influences. Clears and cleanses. Detoxifies the subtle bodies and dissipates energy blockages. Associated with the cougar in the animal kingdom.

MARCH 22

Aromatic affirmation with Juniper Berry

Sit quietly. Close your eyes. Take three slow, relaxed, deep breaths. Open your eyes. Put a drop of Juniper Berry on a tissue and inhale the aroma through your nose. Pause and inhale again. Say out loud or internally the following affirmation: "I am protected. I am whole and present."

Juniper Berry helps to protect you from negative influences so that you can be completely present.

Aromatic emotional self-discovery with Juniper Berry

Sit quietly. Close your eyes. Take three slow, relaxed, deep breaths. Open your eyes. Put a drop of Juniper Berry on a tissue and inhale the aroma through your nose. Pause and inhale again. Ask yourself the following questions and jot down your answers and reflections on a piece of paper.

- ⤙ What negativity is currently affecting me (such as from relationships, work, the environment, and so on)?
- ⤙ How is this negativity manifesting itself in my behavior?
- ⤙ How do I experience this negativity in my body (such as stomachache), mind (such as inability to concentrate), and heart (such as being unkind)?
- ⤙ What negativity am I ready to release?
- ⤙ How will I benefit from being without this negativity?

Inhale the aroma of Juniper Berry again. As you exhale through your mouth, sigh out loud, drop your shoulders, and let go of all the negativity you can. Inhale the aroma one more time. On the exhale, image a shield of light around you, protecting you from negative influences.

Juniper Berry helps to protect you from negativity, as well as clear it away.

Aromatic manifesting ceremony with Juniper Berry

Sit quietly. Close your eyes. Take three slow, relaxed, deep breaths. Open your eyes. Find an object that represents "protection" for you, such as a picture of the archangel Michael, a special stone, a piece of jewelry, or an article of clothing. Set it in front of you. Put a drop of Juniper Berry on a tissue and inhale the aroma through your nose. Pause and inhale again. Hold your hands over or around the object as you send the intention of protection into the object. From now on, whenever you see, touch, wear, or remember this object, the sense of being protected will be with you in body, mind, heart, and spirit. If you choose, place the object in a special place as a reminder.

Juniper Berry helps to protect you against harmful, negative influences.

Aromatic blessing with Juniper Berry

Sit quietly. Close your eyes. Take three slow, relaxed, deep breaths. Open your eyes. Put a drop of Juniper Berry on a tissue and inhale the aroma through your nose. Pause and inhale again. Say out loud or internally: "Bless my body—may I be healthy and protected. Bless my mind—may I be at peace and protected. Bless my heart—may I be loving and protected. Bless my spirit—may I be enlightened and protected."

Juniper Berry helps to protect you from negative influences in every dimension of your being.

Aromatic activity with Juniper Berry

While standing comfortably with your feet slightly apart, close your eyes. Take three slow, relaxed, deep breaths. Open your eyes. Put a drop of Juniper Berry on two pieces of tissue and hold a piece in each hand with your fingertips. Put your hands side by side and inhale the aroma through your nose. Pause and inhale again. Now, begin moving your hands around your body to envelop it in the aroma of Juniper Berry. Move them in front of you, to the right, to the left, above your head, and around your head. Reach behind you as far as you comfortably can. Lift each foot and move your hands around them. You are creating a bubble of protection, as strong as you need it to be. This protection allows all that is positive to come in, and all that is negative to stay out.

Juniper Berry helps to create protection around you that allows in what is positive and keeps out what is negative.

Aromatic visualization with Juniper Berry

Sit quietly. Close your eyes. Take three slow, relaxed, deep breaths. Open your eyes. Put a drop of Juniper Berry on a tissue and inhale the aroma through your nose. Pause and inhale again. Close your eyes. Visualize a beautiful garden.

Experience it completely. See the beauty, smell the aromas, feel the air, and hear the sounds. You want to protect this beauty—this sanctuary. Inhale the aroma of Juniper Berry again. As you do, decide what kind of protection will be best for this garden. It might be a wall, a fence, or a dome. Experiment and discover which protection feels just right, and put it in place. Affirm that this is a special garden and that it is now protected. Everything that happens here is dedicated to its well-being. Imagine how this applies to you. Intend that you are well-protected and all that influences you is for your well-being.

Juniper Berry helps to create and hold a protective barrier that meets your needs and intentions.

MARCH 28
Aromatic prayer with Juniper Berry

Sit quietly. Close your eyes. Take three slow, relaxed, deep breaths. Open your eyes. Put a drop of Juniper Berry on a tissue and inhale the aroma through your nose. Pause and inhale again. Pray out loud or internally: "Great Protector, guard me from negativity and keep my gentle spirit ever in Your safe hands. May I shine brightly so that I might be of greater service to You. Amen."

Juniper Berry helps to protect you from the spiritual darkness of negativity, so that you may be a bright light in the world.

End-of-the-Month Days

Write an aromatic affirmation for cleansing and releasing

In a small glass container, mix together:

> 2 drops Lemongrass to clear and cleanse
> 6 drops Grapefruit to release negative emotions
> 4 drops Juniper Berry to protect against negativity

Have a pen and paper ready. Sit quietly. Close your eyes. Take three slow, relaxed, deep breaths. Open your eyes. Put a drop of your blend on a tissue and inhale the aroma through your nose. Pause and inhale again. Prepare to write an affirmation for cleansing and releasing. Identify what it is that you intend to cleanse away and release. Now write a positive statement about you that describes having already achieved that intention in body, mind, heart, and spirit, as if it is already a reality—for example, "I am free of jealousy and its negative effects." Allow your affirmation to come sincerely from within. Be as specific as possible. Read it out loud and put it in a place to see throughout the day. Read it often today.

Aromatic clearing activity for your home

Sit quietly. Close your eyes. Take three slow, relaxed, deep breaths. Open your eyes. Put a drop of Lemongrass on a

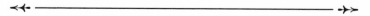

tissue and inhale the aroma through your nose. Pause and inhale again. Stand up and go from room to room, removing one item from each room. Set each item aside and intend to give it to someone, donate it, recycle it, or dispose of it. Excess clutter in your home hinders your energy and creativity. Weather permitting, open all the windows and let a fresh breeze clear away stagnant air and reenergize your home.

Aromatic ceremony to honor Spring

Make a blend to honor Spring. In a small glass container, mix together:

> 1 drop Lemongrass to clear and cleanse
> 4 drops Mandarin for optimism
> 3 drops Bergamot for hope
> 3 drops Coriander for creativity
> 1 drop Nutmeg for new beginnings

Gather together four small planting pots and enough soil to fill them. Choose four seeds or seedlings of plants you would enjoy growing this season. Sit quietly. Close your eyes. Take three slow, relaxed, deep breaths. Open your eyes. Put a drop of your blend on a tissue and inhale the aroma through your nose. Pause and inhale again. Open your eyes and determine four intentions for this Spring: 1) Identify a new perspective you want to embrace. 2) Name a feeling you would like to experience. 3) Think of a healthy habit you want to form. 4) Discover something that would enhance your spirituality. Write them down, such as:

1. I will be positive in all situations, as best I can. (new perspective)

2. I am a joyful person. (feeling)

3. I will drink tea instead of soda. (habit)

4. I choose to surrender and trust in Spirit. (spirituality)

Now, choose a seed/seedling to plant in the first pot, and as you do, say your first intention out loud. Choose another to plant for your second intention, and so on. Water them, knowing that you are nurturing your intentions. Place the pots in a sunny, warm place, aware that you are bringing to these plants, and to yourself, all that is needed to "grow" these intentions this Spring. Every time you tend to these plants and watch them grow, be aware of how these new patterns are flourishing in your body, mind, heart, and spirit.

Inhale your aromatherapy blend again and know that you are fully supported in what you are "planting" for yourself this Spring.

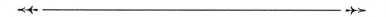

⭐ April ⭐

April is the second Spring month—a time to open your heart to the joy of being alive. It is the time to embrace optimism and hope for the present and the future. The essential oils for this month are Orange for joy, Mandarin for optimism, Petitgrain for harmonious relationships, and Bergamot for hope.

Orange
Best essential oil for joy.

> *Joy is not in things; it is in us.*
> –Richard Wagner

LATIN NAME: *Citrus sinensis*

EXTRACTED FROM: Fruit rind

PSYCHOLOGICAL PROPERTIES: Uplifts. Eases minor depression. Eases stress and tension. Relieves boredom and worry.

SUBTLE PROPERTIES: Promotes joy and delight. Brings in positive energy with its "sunlight" quality. Associated with the hummingbird in the animal kingdom.

APRIL 1
Aromatic affirmation with Orange

Sit quietly. Close your eyes. Take three slow, relaxed, deep breaths. Open your eyes. Put a drop of Orange on a tissue and inhale the aroma through your nose. Pause and inhale again. Say out loud or internally the following affirmation: "I am joyful It is wonderful to be alive."

Orange helps you to discover and experience the joy that is in your life, here and now.

APRIL 2
Aromatic emotional self-discovery with Orange
Sit quietly. Close your eyes. Take three slow, relaxed, deep breaths. Open your eyes. Put a drop of Orange on a tissue and inhale the aroma through your nose. Pause and inhale again. Ask yourself the following questions and jot down your answers on a piece of paper.

- What does "joy" mean to me?
- What areas of my life bring me joy?
- In what areas of my life do I give joy?
- Do I notice and make the most of opportunities for joy? If not, why not?
- How do I benefit from joy?

Inhale the aroma of Orange again and imagine that you are breathing in a sense of joy. Review your answers to the above questions. Reflect and jot down any additional notes.

Orange helps you to experience joy and to identify opportunities in your life to be joyous. It also helps you bring joy to others.

APRIL 3
Aromatic clearing ceremony with Orange

While standing comfortably with your feet slightly apart, close your eyes. Take three slow, relaxed, deep breaths. Open your eyes. Put a drop of Orange on a tissue and inhale the aroma through your nose. Pause and inhale again. With your dominant hand, make three counterclockwise (up on the left, down on the right) circles in front of your forehead, then your heart, and lastly, your stomach area, without touching. Raise your hand in front of your mouth and blow forcefully across your palm with the intention that you are releasing all that interferes with your being able to experience joy. Inhale Orange again. Feel yourself free to feel and embrace joy.

Orange helps you to clear away and release what prevents you from experiencing joy.

APRIL 4
Aromatic blessing with Orange

Sit quietly. Close your eyes. Take three slow, relaxed, deep breaths. Open your eyes. Put a drop of Orange on a tissue and inhale the aroma through your nose. Pause and inhale again. Create a blessing in which you name and bless the things that bring you joy in your life, both large and small. Say out loud or internally: "Bless _____ for the joy it brings to my life." When you are finished naming as many things as you like, end with, "I give thanks for all the joy that blesses my life."

Orange helps you to experience and know the blessing of joy in your life.

APRIL 5
Aromatic activity with Orange

Sit quietly. Close your eyes. Take three slow, relaxed, deep breaths. Open your eyes. Put a drop of Orange on a tissue and inhale the aroma through your nose. Pause and inhale again. Think about what you can do today that will bring joy to someone. It can be someone who you know, such as a friend, or do not know, such as a clerk in a store. You might send a note of gratitude or a bouquet of flowers. You could help with chores or run an errand. You might simply give them a compliment. Intend that you will accomplish this today and then set out to do so.

Orange helps you to experience joy and naturally share it with others.

APRIL 6
Aromatic visualization with Orange

Sit quietly. Close your eyes. Take three slow, relaxed, deep breaths. Open your eyes. Put a drop of Orange on a tissue and inhale the aroma through your nose. Pause and inhale again. Visualize a beautiful garden. Look at the sky and notice the magnificence of the sun. Become aware of the sunlight and how it generously permeates and nourishes everything in this garden. Feel its power and expanse. Sense the garden filling with joy and delight as it basks in the sunlight's splendor. Sense your body enveloped and saturated with this joyful radiance and be aware of the joy that is within you as it unfolds and ever expands.

Orange helps you to experience joy and grow ever more joyful.

APRIL 7
Aromatic prayer with Orange
Sit quietly. Close your eyes. Take three slow, relaxed, deep breaths. Open your eyes. Put a drop of Orange on a tissue and inhale the aroma through your nose. Pause and inhale again. Pray out loud or internally: "May this be a time of joy awakening in my body, mind, heart, and spirit. May I find joy, even in the smallest details of my life. May I experience joy each and every day, and share it with others in Your name. Amen."

Orange helps you to experience joy every day, in all things, and to embrace the opportunities to share it, in alignment with the Divine.

Mandarin

Best essential oil for optimism.

> *Optimism is the faith that leads*
> *to achievement. Nothing can be done*
> *without hope and confidence.*
> –Helen Keller

LATIN NAME: *Citrus reticulata var. mandarin*

EXTRACTED FROM: Fruit rind

PSYCHOLOGICAL PROPERTIES: Relaxes. Relieves anxiety, tension, and stress. Eases restlessness.

SUBTLE PROPERTIES: Promotes optimism and encourages rediscovery of childlike optimism and exuberance. Associated with the dolphin in the animal kingdom.

APRIL 8
Aromatic affirmation with Mandarin

Sit quietly. Close your eyes. Take three slow, relaxed, deep breaths. Open your eyes. Put a drop of Mandarin on a tissue and inhale the aroma through your nose. Pause and inhale again. Say out loud or internally the following affirmation: "My optimistic and playful inner child is alive and well."

Mandarin helps you to experience childlike optimism and exuberance.

Aromatic emotional self-discovery with Mandarin

Sit quietly. Close your eyes. Take three slow, relaxed, deep breaths. Open your eyes. Put a drop of Mandarin on a tissue and inhale the aroma through your nose. Pause and inhale again. Ask yourself the following questions and jot down your answers and reflections on a piece of paper.

- What does "childlike optimism" mean to me?
- What helps me believe in the goodness of life?
- What did I love to do as a child?
- What qualities of the child do I long for in my life now?
- What can I do to incorporate these qualities into my life now?
- How will reconnecting with childhood optimism benefit me?

Inhale the aroma of Mandarin again and intend that you are breathing in childlike optimism and enthusiasm. Review your answers to the above questions. Reflect and jot down any additional notes.

Mandarin helps you to remember and reconnect with the optimism and enthusiasm of childhood.

APRIL 10
Aromatic attracting ceremony with Mandarin

Sit quietly. Close your eyes. Take three slow, relaxed, deep breaths. Open your eyes. Put a drop of Mandarin on a tissue and inhale the aroma through your nose. Pause and inhale again. Light a candle. As you look at the candle, experience its radiant light filling your body, mind, heart, and spirit with optimism. Allow it to permeate your entire being. Inhale Mandarin from the tissue once again. Feel the gentle clearing away of anything that prevents you from having an optimistic attitude. Feel yourself radiating the bright light of optimism.

Mandarin helps you to be optimistic and cheerful, and to send these qualities out to the world.

APRIL 11
Aromatic blessing with Mandarin

Sit quietly. Close your eyes. Take three slow, relaxed, deep breaths. Open your eyes. Put a drop of Mandarin on a tissue and inhale the aroma through your nose. Pause and inhale again. Say out loud or internally: "Bless the experiences of my inner child. Bless the expressions of my inner child. Bless the optimistic, enthusiastic, and happy child within me."

Mandarin helps you to experience and express childlike optimism in your life.

Aromatic activity with Mandarin

Sit quietly. Close your eyes. Take three slow, relaxed, deep breaths. Open your eyes. Put a drop of Mandarin on a tissue and inhale the aroma through your nose. Pause and inhale again. Sit or stand comfortably and imagine your happy inner child coming forth. Feel the exuberant, playful, creative, and optimistic energy in your body. Reacquaint yourself with any aspect of this feeling that is unfamiliar. Take some time to become comfortable with this experience. Now, move your body in a way that expresses this energy, such as dancing, jumping, or skipping. Remember to use these physical expressions whenever you want to experience this aspect of your inner child.

Mandarin helps you to embody the happy, playful inner child.

Aromatic visualization with Mandarin

Sit quietly. Close your eyes. Take three slow, relaxed, deep breaths. Open your eyes. Put a drop of Mandarin on a tissue and inhale the aroma through your nose. Pause and inhale again. Visualize a beautiful garden. As you look around, bring forth and engage the senses of sight, hearing, smell, and touch. Experience this garden in new, childlike ways. Decide if there is anything you would like to bring here such as a swing set, a sandbox, plants, rocks, bridges, or benches. Become a creative, enthusiastic landscape designer. In your imagination, begin playing in the garden. Play with making changes—moving things around or adding new things. Experiment and have fun.

Mandarin helps allow you to play and experiment, just for the fun of it.

Aromatic prayer with Mandarin

Sit quietly. Close your eyes. Take three slow, relaxed, deep breaths. Open your eyes. Put a drop of Mandarin on a tissue and inhale the aroma through your nose. Pause and inhale again. Pray out loud or internally: "May the Divine Child within me awaken optimism and exuberance in my body, mind, heart, and spirit. Amen."

Mandarin helps you to experience childlike optimism that is divinely inspired.

Petitgrain

Best essential oil for harmonious relationships.

> *Treasure your relationships,*
> *not your possessions.*
> –Anthony J. D'Angelo

LATIN NAME: *Citrus aurantium var. amara*

EXTRACTED FROM: Fruit rind

PSYCHOLOGICAL PROPERTIES: Calms. Refreshes. Promotes mental clarity. Relieves mental fatigue. Eases anger.

SUBTLE PROPERTIES: Promotes harmony, especially in relationships. Promotes a healthy self-esteem. Brings in positive energy. Associated with the archangel Raguel in the angelic realm and the horse in the animal kingdom.

APRIL 15
Aromatic affirmation with Petitgrain

Sit quietly. Close your eyes. Take three slow, relaxed, deep breaths. Open your eyes. Put a drop of Petitgrain on a tissue and inhale the aroma through your nose. Pause and inhale again. Say out loud or internally the following affirmation: "The harmony within me promotes harmony in my life and in all my relationships."

Petitgrain helps you to experience harmony in your life, with yourself, and with others.

Aromatic emotional self-discovery with Petitgrain

Sit quietly. Close your eyes. Take three slow, relaxed, deep breaths. Open your eyes. Put a drop of Petitgrain on a tissue and inhale the aroma through your nose. Pause and inhale again. Ask yourself the following questions and jot down your answers and reflections on a piece of paper.

- ⤳ What does a "harmonious relationship" mean to me?
- ⤳ Which of my relationships are harmonious?
- ⤳ Which of my relationships are not harmonious?
- ⤳ How does disharmony feel to me?
- ⤳ What can I do to promote more harmony in my relationships?
- ⤳ How will I benefit from having harmonious relationships?

Inhale the aroma of Petitgrain again and intend that you are breathing in a sense of harmony. Review your answers to the above questions. Reflect and jot down any additional notes.

Petitgrain helps you to experience harmony in your relationships and to recognize the sources of harmony and disharmony.

Aromatic integrating ceremony with Petitgrain

Sit quietly. Close your eyes. Take three slow, relaxed, deep breaths. Open your eyes. Put a drop of Petitgrain on a tissue and inhale the aroma through your nose. Pause and inhale again. Pour some water into a glass. Hold the glass of water with both hands and intend that it is imbued with light and the ability to have healthy and harmonious relationships in your life. Drink the water. As you do, think: "I am filled with light that brings harmony to all my relationships." When you have finished drinking, experience the feeling that there will be positive shifts, as needed, in your relationships in the future.

Petitgrain helps you to bring harmony to your relationships.

Aromatic blessing with Petitgrain

Sit quietly. Close your eyes. Take three slow, relaxed, deep breaths. Open your eyes. Put a drop of Petitgrain on a tissue and inhale the aroma through your nose. Pause and inhale again. Say out loud or internally: "I bless all of my relationships. I bless all of the people with whom I am connected. May my relationships be blessed with harmony and peace."

Petitgrain helps you to experience the blessings of harmonious relationships.

Aromatic activity with Petitgrain

Sit quietly. Close your eyes. Take three slow, relaxed, deep breaths. Open your eyes. Put a drop of Petitgrain on a tissue and inhale the aroma through your nose. Pause and inhale again. Cut three pieces of string or ribbon twelve inches in length. Secure them together at one end with tape or a rubber band, or by tying them in a knot. Think of a relationship to which you intend to bring harmony, and name the person out loud. Carefully braid the three strands. As you do, be aware that you are weaving together yourself, the other person, and the spirit of harmony. Carry this braid with you for one week as a reminder.

Petitgrain helps you to bring harmony into specific relationships.

Aromatic visualization with Petitgrain

Sit quietly. Close your eyes. Take three slow, relaxed, deep breaths. Open your eyes. Put a drop of Petitgrain on a tissue and inhale the aroma through your nose. Pause and inhale again. Visualize a beautiful garden. Look around on the ground and notice that there are a variety of seeds lying there. Imagine the appearance of these seeds. Are they small or large, furry or smooth, light or dark? Notice the ones to which you are drawn and pick up five of them. Why were you drawn to them? What was it about these seeds that you liked? Do they represent a particular quality? How do these seeds harmonize with each other? How do they harmonize with the garden? Notice the qualities that are important to you. Place the seeds in a safe place, knowing that you will plant them when the time is right.

Petitgrain helps you to experience harmony and make choices that promote harmony in your life.

APRIL 21
Aromatic prayer with Petitgrain

Sit quietly. Close your eyes. Take three slow, relaxed, deep breaths. Open your eyes. Put a drop of Petitgrain on a tissue and inhale the aroma through your nose. Pause and inhale again. Pray out loud or internally: "Dear God, just as You offer Yourself to me in loving relationship, may I, with Your grace and blessing, offer myself to others in loving harmony. I ask that You help me to be in harmony with all sentient beings—people, animals, plants, and Mother Earth. Amen."

Petitgrain helps you to experience harmonious, loving relationships with the support of the Divine.

Bergamot

Best essential oil for hope.

> *Hope is a waking dream.*
> –Aristotle

LATIN NAME: *Citrus bergamia*

Expressed from: Fruit rind

PSYCHOLOGICAL PROPERTIES: Uplifts and calms. Refreshes. Eases anxiety and mild depression. Relieves anger and frustration.

SUBTLE PROPERTIES: Promotes hope. Brings in positive energy—light into dark times. Lightens a heavy or wounded heart. Helps the heart to radiate love. Promotes joy. Associated with the penguin in the animal kingdom.

APRIL 22
Aromatic affirmation with Bergamot

Sit quietly. Close your eyes. Take three slow, relaxed, deep breaths. Open your eyes. Put a drop of Bergamot on a tissue and inhale the aroma through your nose. Pause and inhale again. Say out loud or internally the following affirmation: "I commit to being hopeful in my thoughts, words, and deeds in simple and practical ways."

Bergamot helps you to experience and embrace hope as an active principle by which to live.

Aromatic emotional self-discovery with Bergamot

Sit quietly. Close your eyes. Take three slow, relaxed, deep breaths. Open your eyes. Put a drop of Bergamot on a tissue and inhale the aroma through your nose. Pause and inhale again. Ask yourself the following questions and jot down your answers and reflections on a piece of paper.

> ⤚ What does "hope" mean to me?
> ⤚ Do I experience hope in my life?
> ⤚ What do I hope for?
> ⤚ Is there anything I am unable to be hopeful about? What is it?
> ⤚ What discourages my being hopeful?
> ⤚ How can I be more hopeful?
> ⤚ How does being hopeful benefit me?

Inhale the aroma of Bergamot again and intend that you are breathing in a sense of hope. Review your answers to the above questions. Reflect and jot down any additional notes.

Bergamot helps you to experience and understand the virtue of hope in your life.

APRIL 24
Aromatic manifesting ceremony with Bergamot

Sit quietly. Close your eyes. Take three slow, relaxed, deep breaths. Open your eyes. Find or create an object that represents "hope" for you, such as an angel statue, a special stone, a picture of a person, or a favorite book. Set it in front of you. Put a drop of Bergamot on a tissue and inhale the aroma through your nose. Pause and inhale again. Hold your hands over or around the object as you send the intention of hope into the object. From now on, whenever you see, touch, or remember that object, the sense of being hopeful will be with you in body, mind, heart, and spirit. If you choose, place the object in a special place as a reminder.

Bergamot helps to bring the good qualities of hope into your consciousness and life.

Aromatic blessing with Bergamot

Sit quietly. Close your eyes. Take three slow, relaxed, deep breaths. Open your eyes. Put a drop of Bergamot on a tissue and inhale the aroma through your nose. Pause and inhale again. Say out loud or internally: "I bless all the sources of hope in my life and all of the opportunities to be hopeful. I bless the people in my life who help me to be hopeful. I bless all that I hope for—may it come to pass for the good of all."

Bergamot helps you to experience being hopeful, reminding you to bless and cherish what nurtures and sustains your sense of hope.

Aromatic activity with Bergamot

Sit quietly. Close your eyes. Take three slow, relaxed, deep breaths. Open your eyes. Put a drop of Bergamot on a tissue and inhale the aroma through your nose. Pause and inhale again. Remember a time when you experienced a strong sense of hope. Remember how it felt to you. Now draw that feeling into your stomach, heart, and throat areas. Imagine what it would sound like if it were expressed in a song. Imagine what it would look like if it were expressed in dance. If you are comfortable in doing so, express your experience of hope with a song and/or a dance. Notice how it reverberates throughout your body, when expressed in these ways. Notice what it feels like to embody a sense of hope.

Bergamot helps to fill you with hope and allows you to express it in what you say and do.

APRIL 27
Aromatic visualization with Bergamot

Sit quietly. Close your eyes. Take three slow, relaxed, deep breaths. Open your eyes. Put a drop of Bergamot on a tissue and inhale the aroma through your nose. Pause and inhale again. Visualize a small plot of ground that has been prepared for a garden. Choose a wide variety of flower seeds to plant. What types of flowers have you chosen? What size are they? What color are they? What are their other qualities? Plant them exactly where you would like them to be. Carefully tend to these seeds. Protect and nurture them. Water them and know that you have planted the seeds of hope and beauty. Look forward to watching this garden grow. Look forward to these qualities growing in you.

Bergamot helps you to experience hope and to nurture the practice of hope in your life.

Aromatic prayer with Bergamot

Sit quietly. Close your eyes. Take three slow, relaxed, deep breaths. Open your eyes. Put a drop of Bergamot on a tissue and inhale the aroma through your nose. Pause and inhale again. Pray out loud or internally: "Great Creator, Your overflowing love bountifully fills my life. Plant the virtue of hope in my soul and spirit. May my practice of hope help me to grow in Your service. Amen."

Bergamot helps you to experience hope as a spiritual practice.

End-of-the-Month Days

APRIL 29
Write an aromatic affirmation for hope and optimism

In a small glass container, mix together:

> 2 drops Mandarin for optimism
> 5 drops Bergamot for hope
> 5 drops Orange for joy

Have a pen and paper ready. Sit quietly. Close your eyes. Take three slow, relaxed, deep breaths. Open your eyes. Put a drop of your blend on a tissue and inhale the aroma through your nose. Pause and inhale again. Prepare to write an affirmation for hope and optimism. Identify what it is you are intending to be hopeful and optimistic about. Write a positive statement about yourself that describes what you desire in body, mind, heart, and spirit, as if it is already a reality—for example, "I have the perfect job." Allow your affirmation to come sincerely from within. Be as specific as possible. Read it out loud and put it in a place to see throughout the day. Read it often today.

APRIL 30
Aromatic activity for creative goals

Sit quietly. Close your eyes. Take three slow, relaxed, deep breaths. Open your eyes. Put a drop of Coriander on a tissue

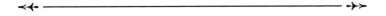

and inhale the aroma through your nose. Pause and inhale again. Get a pen and paper. On the top, write "Creative Goals" and draw lines to divide the page into four columns. Across the top, entitle the first column "Body," the second column "Mind," the third column "Heart," and the fourth column "Spirit." In each column, write one to three goals you have for yourself for that theme. Inhale Coriander once again and imagine how your life will be when these goals are achieved. Become aware that all of these goals are coming together as one. Each time you take a step in accomplishing one, creative energy is generated to pursue and accomplish another. Place your list in a place where you can see it and reflect upon it. As you accomplish your goals, take the time to alter and rework the list so it evolves as you evolve.

◄◄─ ─── ─►►

⤛ May ⤜

May is the third and last Spring month—a time to be receptive to, as well as initiate, new beginnings. It is a time of rebirth and inspiration, and for creative expression to find fertile soil. The essential oils for this month are Geranium to support the feminine, Coriander for creativity, Nutmeg to support new beginnings, Eucalyptus for inspiration, and Mimosa for renewal.

Geranium

Best essential oil to support the feminine. Embodies the spirit of Spring.

> *There can be no spirituality,*
> *no sanctity, no truth without*
> *the female sex.*
> –Diane Frolov and Andrew Schneider

LATIN NAME: *Pelargonium graveolens*

EXTRACTED FROM: Flowering plant

PSYCHOLOGICAL PROPERTIES: Tones the nervous system. Helps balance moods/emotions. Eases anxiety and depression.

SUBTLE PROPERTIES: Supports and nurtures the feminine. Promotes receptivity and creativity. Inspires. Supports new beginnings and rebirth. Associated with the swan in the animal kingdom.

Aromatic affirmation with Geranium

Sit quietly. Close your eyes. Take three slow, relaxed, deep breaths. Open your eyes. Put a drop of Geranium on a tissue and inhale the aroma through your nose. Pause and inhale again. Say out loud or internally the following affirmation: "I embrace the feminine. I am nurturing, receptive, and creative. I act with wisdom and love."

Geranium helps you to embrace the feminine and its wise, nurturing, receptive, and creative qualities.

Aromatic emotional self-discovery with Geranium

Sit quietly. Close your eyes. Take three slow, relaxed, deep breaths. Open your eyes. Put a drop of Geranium on a tissue and inhale the aroma through your nose. Pause and inhale again. Ask yourself the following questions and jot down your answers and reflections on a piece of paper.

- What does "the feminine" mean to me? What are its qualities?
- How do I experience the feminine in my life?
- Are there ways in which I embrace the feminine? If so, what are they?
- Are there ways in which I ignore or negatively judge the feminine? If so, what are they?
- How does embracing the feminine benefit me?

Inhale the aroma of Geranium again and intend that you are breathing in the qualities of the feminine. Review your answers to the above questions. Reflect and jot down any additional notes.

Geranium helps you to embrace and understand the qualities of the feminine.

MAY 3
Aromatic clearing ceremony with Geranium

While standing comfortably with your feet slightly apart, close your eyes. Take three slow, relaxed, deep breaths. Open your eyes. Put a drop of Geranium on a tissue and inhale the aroma through your nose. Pause and inhale again. With your dominant hand, make three counterclockwise (up on the left, down on the right) circles in front of your forehead, then your heart, and lastly, your stomach area, without touching. Then raise your hand in front of your mouth and blow forcefully across your palm with the intention that you are clearing away and releasing any negative thoughts, feelings, or beliefs regarding the power, integrity, and qualities pertaining to the feminine. Inhale Geranium again and feel supported and inspired to embrace the feminine.

Geranium helps you to experience the qualities of the feminine and to release any negativity and misunderstanding you have about them.

MAY 4
Aromatic blessing with Geranium

Sit quietly. Close your eyes. Take three slow, relaxed, deep breaths. Open your eyes. Put a drop of Geranium on a tissue and inhale the aroma through your nose. Pause and inhale again. Say out loud or internally: "Bless this time of rebirth and new beginnings. Bless the gentle qualities of Spring and all the ways in which I dream and prepare for starting anew."

Geranium embodies the essence of Spring and supports you in times of "new beginnings."

MAY 5
Aromatic activity with Geranium

Sit quietly. Close your eyes. Take three slow, relaxed, deep breaths. Open your eyes. Put a drop of Geranium on a tissue and inhale the aroma through your nose. Pause and inhale again. Gently rest your hands on your stomach and slightly bow your head, with your eyes closed. Take a long, slow, deep breath followed by a long, slow exhale. Slowly open your eyes and gradually lift your head, looking upward. Open your arms wide, out to the sides, reaching and opening to the heavens. Remain in this position of being "open and receptive" for as long as you are comfortable. With each breath, feel yourself being "open" to and inspired for new beginnings and a new way of living.

Geranium helps you to experience being open and receptive to new beginnings and positive changes.

Aromatic visualization with Geranium

Sit quietly. Close your eyes. Take three slow, relaxed, deep breaths. Open your eyes. Put a drop of Geranium on a tissue and inhale the aroma through your nose. Pause and inhale again. Visualize a beautiful garden. As you explore this garden, notice that you are drawn to a natural cavern. Approach it, and as you do, become aware that this area is dedicated to the feminine and its revered qualities. What is in this area? Are there statues? Stones? Plants? Flowers? Animals? What do these items reveal to you about the feminine? How do you feel? Is there anything you would like to change or add? Create this place exactly as you would like it to be—in honor of the sacred feminine and your understanding of it. Imagine that something in you is naturally shifting in a positive way. Step back and enjoy the beauty of the area you have created.

Geranium helps you to experience and honor the feminine.

Aromatic prayer with Geranium

Sit quietly. Close your eyes. Take three slow, relaxed, deep breaths. Open your eyes. Put a drop of Geranium on a tissue and inhale the aroma through your nose. Pause and inhale again. Pray out loud or internally: "Dear Mother Earth, help me be open and receptive, as you are, to new life and new beginnings. Gently prepare me so that I might experience this gift. Help me to receive only what is for my highest good. Amen."

Geranium helps you to begin anew and receive in ways that support your highest good.

Coriander

Best essential oil for creativity.

> *All the works of man*
> *have their origin in creative fantasy.*
> –Carl Jung

LATIN NAME: *Coriandrum sativum*

EXTRACTED FROM: Seeds

PSYCHOLOGICAL PROPERTIES: Uplifts and refreshes the mind. Has mild euphoric properties. Relieves fatigue, tension, and lethargy.

SUBTLE PROPERTIES: Encourages creativity and creative expression. Promotes spontaneity and imagination. Associated with the beaver in the animal kingdom.

MAY 8
Aromatic affirmation with Coriander

Sit quietly. Close your eyes. Take three slow, relaxed, deep breaths. Open your eyes. Put a drop of Coriander on a tissue and inhale the aroma through your nose. Pause and inhale again. Say out loud or internally the following affirmation: "I am creative. I express myself with creativity and imagination."

Coriander helps you to experience creativity and imagination, and to express yourself creatively.

Aromatic emotional self-discovery with Coriander

Sit quietly. Close your eyes. Take three slow, relaxed, deep breaths. Open your eyes. Put a drop of Coriander on a tissue and inhale the aroma through your nose. Pause and inhale again. Ask yourself the following questions and jot down your answers and reflections on a piece of paper.

> ⤙ What does "being creative" mean to me?
> ⤙ In what areas of my life am I creative?
> ⤙ In what areas of my life do I feel I lack creativity?
> ⤙ What would I like to create?
> ⤙ How does being creative benefit me?

Inhale the aroma of Coriander again and intend that you are breathing in the ability to be creative. Review your answers to the above questions. Reflect and jot down any additional notes.

Coriander helps you to explore creativity and identify how you experience it in your life.

Aromatic attracting ceremony with Coriander

Sit quietly. Close your eyes. Take three slow, relaxed, deep breaths. Open your eyes. Put a drop of Coriander on a tissue and inhale the aroma through your nose. Pause and inhale again. Light a candle. As you look at the candle, experience its radiant light filling you with creativity, spontaneity, and imagination. Let it fill your body, mind, heart, and spirit. Feel it permeate your entire being. Once again, inhale Coriander. Feel yourself embodying and radiating endless creativity.

Coriander helps you to embody the expansive qualities of creativity.

Aromatic blessing with Coriander

Sit quietly. Close your eyes. Take three slow, relaxed, deep breaths. Open your eyes. Put a drop of Coriander on a tissue and inhale the aroma through your nose. Pause and inhale again. Say out loud or internally the following blessing: "Bless all that helps me to be creative and creatively expressive. Bless and honor all that I am guided to create. May all that I create be for the good of all."

Coriander helps you to be creative and to receive all its blessings.

Aromatic activity with Coriander

Sit quietly. Close your eyes. Take three slow, relaxed, deep breaths. Open your eyes. Put a drop of Coriander on a tissue and inhale the aroma through your nose. Pause and inhale again. Imagine one thing that you could do today to demonstrate your creativity. It could be a large project that you have been waiting to begin, such as making a scrapbook of your photos, or painting a room a new color. It could be a simple thing, such as gathering a bouquet of flowers for the kitchen table, or simply rearranging a few pieces of furniture.

Imagine doing this project and how you feel upon its completion. Imagine how it will affect other people. Now open your eyes and make it your intention to do, or begin, your project today.

Coriander helps you to be creative and supports your creative projects.

MAY 13
Aromatic visualization with Coriander

Sit quietly. Close your eyes. Take three slow, relaxed, deep breaths. Open your eyes. Put a drop of Coriander on a tissue and inhale the aroma through your nose. Pause and inhale again. Visualize a beautiful garden. Become conscious of all your senses—seeing, hearing, smelling, feeling, and even tasting. Bask in the warmth of the Spring sun on your skin. Notice how you relax as you are enveloped in that gentle warmth. Be aware how this light and warmth provide for the creation of new life. Look around and see how the garden receives this warmth. Imagine the warmth gently penetrating the damp earth, and surrounding the seeds and roots of the plants in this garden, encouraging and inspiring new growth. Feel the earth begin to stir and create new life. Imagine how creativity stirs in you.

Coriander helps you to experience and align with the creative, natural cycles of life.

Aromatic prayer with Coriander

Sit quietly. Close your eyes. Take three slow, relaxed, deep breaths. Open your eyes. Put a drop of Coriander on a tissue and inhale the aroma through your nose. Pause and inhale again. Pray out loud or internally: "May I create joyfully, as You create, Great Spirit. Guide me to create what best serves You. Make me an instrument of your creative expression. Amen."

Coriander helps you to create with divine inspiration.

Nutmeg

Best essential oil to support new beginnings.

Vitality shows in not only the ability
to persist but the ability to start over.
–F. Scott Fitzgerald

LATIN NAME: *Myristica fragrans*

EXTRACTED FROM: Fruit

PSYCHOLOGICAL PROPERTIES: Invigorates the mind. Promotes and intensifies dreaming.

SUBTLE PROPERTIES: Provides support for new beginnings, especially for creative endeavors. Diminishes perceived limitations. Encourages a sense of freedom. Promotes visions. Associated with the crow in the animal kingdom.

MAY 15
Aromatic affirmation with Nutmeg

Sit quietly. Close your eyes. Take three slow, relaxed, deep breaths. Open your eyes. Put a drop of Nutmeg on a tissue and inhale the aroma through your nose. Pause and inhale again. Say out loud or internally the following affirmation: "I celebrate my ability to begin anew. I am joyful and free."

Nutmeg encourages you to feel free to pursue and enjoy new beginnings.

Aromatic emotional self-discovery with Nutmeg

Sit quietly. Close your eyes. Take three slow, relaxed, deep breaths. Open your eyes. Put a drop of Nutmeg on a tissue and inhale the aroma through your nose. Pause and inhale again. Ask yourself the following questions and jot down your answers and reflections on a piece of paper.

- What does "new beginnings" mean to me?
- What new beginnings are occurring in my life right now?
- Am I open to new beginnings?
- Are there ways I resist new beginnings?
- What would I like to begin anew?
- How do new beginnings benefit me?

Inhale the aroma of Nutmeg again and intend that you are breathing in the ability to begin anew. Review your answers to the above questions. Reflect and jot down any additional notes.

Nutmeg helps to support new beginnings and helps you understand their dynamics in your life.

MAY 17
Aromatic integrating ceremony with Nutmeg

Sit quietly. Close your eyes. Take three slow, relaxed, deep breaths. Open your eyes. Put a drop of Nutmeg on a tissue and inhale the aroma through your nose. Pause and inhale again. Pour some water into a glass. Hold the glass of water with both hands and intend that it is imbued with light and the ability to have healthy new beginnings. As you drink the water, think: "I am filled with light and limitless possibilities for new beginnings." When you have finished, set the glass down, and imagine yourself filled with the freedom, energy, and vision that enable inspired new beginnings.

Nutmeg helps you to experience and integrate the ability to begin anew.

MAY 18
Aromatic blessing with Nutmeg

Sit quietly. Close your eyes. Take three slow, relaxed, deep breaths. Open your eyes. Put a drop of Nutmeg on a tissue and inhale the aroma through your nose. Pause and inhale again. Say out loud or internally the following blessing: "Bless each tender, new beginning that is gently making itself known to me. Bless my ability to trust in new life. Bless the newness of body, mind, heart, and spirit that is emerging in me now."

Nutmeg helps you to experience and bless all that is newly emerging in your life.

MAY 19
Aromatic activity with Nutmeg

Sit quietly. Close your eyes. Take three slow, relaxed, deep breaths. Open your eyes. Put a drop of Nutmeg on a tissue and inhale the aroma through your nose. Pause and inhale again. On a piece of paper, write down the following: "If today was the first day of my new life I would ..." Then, write down twelve things that come to you. Pick *one* thing on the list and intend to do it, or begin to do it, today. Notice how beginning something important for the life you want feels to you. Notice how the first step—putting your intentions into motion—is vitally important.

Nutmeg supports you to initiate new patterns of thoughts, feelings, and behavior so that you can grow and evolve.

Aromatic visualization with Nutmeg

Sit quietly. Close your eyes. Take three slow, relaxed, deep breaths. Open your eyes. Put a drop of Nutmeg on a tissue and inhale the aroma through your nose. Pause and inhale again. Visualize a beautiful garden. As you enjoy the feeling of the sun's warmth and fresh air, begin looking around this garden and notice the signs of Spring. See the tiny flower buds and the tender green leaves on the trees and bushes. Notice the places in this garden where you have planted seeds, and witness the tiny shoots emerging from the soil. Know that they will be changing and growing daily to achieve their full expression. Experience the aroma of the soil and the way the plants smell in the fresh air. Feel the new life beginning and growing in this beautiful garden.

Nutmeg helps you to experience and understand the cycle of life, as it begins anew.

Aromatic prayer with Nutmeg

Sit quietly. Close your eyes. Take three slow, relaxed, deep breaths. Open your eyes. Put a drop of Nutmeg on a tissue and inhale the aroma through your nose. Pause and inhale again. Pray out loud or internally: "Great Spirit, You who replenishes this planet and nurtures me every day, I give thanks for the life that returns and for the life that begins anew. Help me to begin each day anew, in You. Amen."

Nutmeg helps you to experience a sense of new beginnings, every day, in spirit.

Eucalyptus

Best essential oil for inspiration.

> *The wise person develops his brain,*
> *and opens his mind to the genius*
> *and spirit of the world's great ideas.*
> *He will feel inspired with the purest*
> *and noblest thoughts that have ever*
> *animated the spirit of humanity.*
> –Alfred A. Montapert

LATIN NAME: *Eucalyptus globulus*

EXTRACTED FROM: Leaves

PSYCHOLOGICAL PROPERTIES: Clears the mind. Improves concentration. Cools the emotions.

SUBTLE PROPERTIES: Inspires. Encourages taking a deep breath for new beginnings. Promotes mental and intuitive clarity. Helps to counteract "burnout." Associated with the condor in the animal kingdom.

MAY 22
Aromatic affirmation with Eucalyptus

Sit quietly. Close your eyes. Take three slow, relaxed, deep breaths. Open your eyes. Put a drop of Eucalyptus on a tissue and inhale the aroma through your nose. Pause and inhale again. Say out loud or internally the following affirmation: "With each breath, I draw upon limitless inspiration to guide and support me through life's changes and new beginnings."

Eucalyptus helps you to be deeply and sincerely inspired.

MAY 23
Aromatic emotional self-discovery with Eucalyptus

Sit quietly. Close your eyes. Take three slow, relaxed, deep breaths. Open your eyes. Put a drop of Eucalyptus on a tissue and inhale the aroma through your nose. Pause and inhale again. Ask yourself the following questions and jot down your answers and reflections on a piece of paper.

- What does "inspiration" mean to me?
- How does inspiration feel to me?
- What inspires me?
- What interferes with my being inspired?
- What activities in my life could be more inspired?
- How do I benefit from being inspired?

Inhale the aroma of Eucalyptus again and intend that you are breathing in a sense of inspiration. Review your answers to the above questions. Reflect and jot down any additional notes.

Eucalyptus helps you to experience inspiration and to understand its dynamics in your life.

MAY 24
Aromatic manifesting ceremony with Eucalyptus

Sit quietly. Close your eyes. Take three slow, relaxed, deep breaths. Open your eyes. Find or create an object that represents "inspiration" to you. This might be a picture of something or someone that actually inspires you or something that represents inspiration to you, such as a book. Set it in front of you. Put a drop of Eucalyptus on a tissue and inhale the aroma through your nose. Pause and inhale again. Hold your hands over or around the object as you send the intention of inspiration into it. From now on, whenever you see, touch, or remember that object, the sense of being inspired will be with you in body, mind, heart, and spirit. If you choose, place the object in a special place as a reminder.

Eucalyptus helps you to feel inspired and act with inspiration.

Aromatic blessing with Eucalyptus

Sit quietly. Close your eyes. Take three slow, relaxed, deep breaths. Open your eyes. Put a drop of Eucalyptus on a tissue and inhale the aroma through your nose. Pause and inhale again. Say out loud or internally: "Bless each breath of inspiration that fills my being. Bless each moment of inspiration that energizes me. Bless all the ways inspiration leads me to achieve my highest destiny."

Eucalyptus helps you to experience inspiration with each breath and every step you take on your life's path.

Aromatic activity with Eucalyptus

Sit quietly. Close your eyes. Take three slow, relaxed, deep breaths. Open your eyes. Put a drop of Eucalyptus on a tissue and inhale the aroma through your nose. Pause and inhale again. Focus on each breath you take, without changing the pattern. Notice the parts of your body that move with your breathing, and the order in which they move. Listen carefully to the sound of each breath. Notice that the temperature of the breath you inhale is different from the temperature of the breath you exhale. Be completely present with your breath. On an exhale, drop your shoulders and gently lower your head. As you inhale again, lift your head up and imagine that your breath is entering every cell of your body, creating health and vitality, and filling you with a sense of inspiration.

Eucalyptus helps you to experience inspiration, enhanced by using conscious attention to breath.

MAY 27
Aromatic visualization with Eucalyptus

Sit quietly. Close your eyes. Take three slow, relaxed, deep breaths. Open your eyes. Put a drop of Eucalyptus on a tissue and inhale the aroma through your nose. Pause and inhale again. Visualize a beautiful garden. Look around and notice all that is in this Spring garden. Breathe in its beauty and splendor. Feel your lungs gently expanding as your body, mind, heart, and spirit are slowly and deeply rejuvenated with fresh, clean, pure air. Walk around this garden and be aware of being energized and inspired as you breathe and move in this beautiful place. Notice the clarity of your thoughts.

Notice that your heart is nurtured. Know that you have exactly what you need to live an inspired life.

Eucalyptus helps you to experience inspiration and receive all you need to be inspired.

Aromatic prayer with Eucalyptus

Sit quietly. Close your eyes. Take three slow, relaxed, deep breaths. Open your eyes. Put a drop of Eucalyptus on a tissue and inhale the aroma through your nose. Pause and inhale again. Pray out loud or internally: "Holy Spirit, with each breath I take, let me be inspired by You. Amen."

Eucalyptus helps you to experience divine inspiration.

End-of-the-Month Days

MAY 29
Write an aromatic affirmation for new beginnings

In a small glass container, mix together:

> 3 drops of Nutmeg to support new beginnings
> 8 drops of Coriander for creativity
> 1 drop of Eucalyptus for inspiration

Have a pen and paper ready. Sit quietly. Close your eyes. Take three slow, relaxed, deep breaths. Open your eyes. Put a drop of your blend on a tissue and inhale the aroma through your nose. Pause and inhale again. Prepare to write an affirmation for new beginnings. Identify what is newly beginning now for you. Write a positive statement about yourself that describes the new beginning that you desire in body, mind, heart, and spirit, as if it is already a reality—for example, "I communicate well in my relationships." Allow your affirmation to come sincerely from within. Be as specific as possible. Read it out loud and put it in a place to see throughout the day. Read it often today.

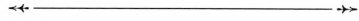

MAY 30
New Spring essential oil: Mimosa

Mimosa

Best essential oil for renewal.

> *We must always change,*
> *renew, rejuvenate ourselves;*
> *otherwise we harden.*
> –Johann Wolfgang von Goethe

LATIN NAME: *Acacia dealbata*

EXTRACTED FROM: Blossoms

PSYCHOLOGICAL PROPERTIES: Soothes and calms. Relieves nervous tension, stress, and anxiety. Eases oversensitivity.

SUBTLE PROPERTIES: Promotes a sense of renewal, youthful attitude, optimism, and delight. Encourages dreaming. Opens the heart to receive love.

Aromatic visualization with Mimosa

Sit quietly. Close your eyes. Take three slow, relaxed, deep breaths. Open your eyes. Put a drop of Mimosa on a tissue and inhale the aroma through your nose. Pause and inhale again. Visualize a gentle vortex spinning out from the core of your body, taking with it and removing the beliefs, thoughts, feelings, or habits that no longer serve you. Allow this spinning to continue until you feel that everything you want to be removed, is removed. Now imagine a golden ball of light twelve inches above your head. Inhale Mimosa again and say internally or out loud: "I call to me now any and all of my energy and youthful attitude, from the past, present, or future. I am ready to be delightfully renewed." Imagine this energy filling the gold ball and then allow the ball to open at its base and gently and slowly pour all of the energy into you, replenishing and renewing you in body, mind, heart, and spirit.

Mimosa helps to renew your energy and encourages a youthful attitude.

MAY 31
Aromatic ceremony to honor your accomplishments this Spring

Choose one of your favorite Spring essential oils: Lemongrass, Bay St. Thomas, Grapefruit, Juniper Berry, Orange, Mandarin, Petitgrain, Bergamot, Mimosa, Geranium, Coriander, Nutmeg, or Eucalyptus. Sit quietly. Close your eyes. Take three slow, relaxed, deep breaths. Open your eyes. Put a drop of your chosen oil on a tissue and inhale the aroma through your nose. Pause and inhale again. Reflect back upon the past Spring season and identify your accomplishments. Don't be modest. Notice each and every goal that you have accomplished, from the smallest to the largest. Inhale your oil once again, and take a large step forward. As you do, say out loud or internally, "I have accomplished _____ this Spring." Inhale your oil again, and take another step, saying out loud or internally, "I have also accomplished _____ in these last few months." With one more step and one final inhalation, say out loud or internally, "I want to be sure I acknowledge accomplishing _____." Now turn around and visualize looking back at yourself prior to taking these three steps. Notice how, in only a few minutes, something has changed within you simply through the process of acknowledging what you have accomplished. Now ask yourself what you might like to do to celebrate what you have accomplished. This could be going for a swim in the ocean or a lake, calling a dear friend, or having a massage. Think of something that would please you and make a commitment to do this for yourself now, to honor your accomplishments this Spring.

Summer

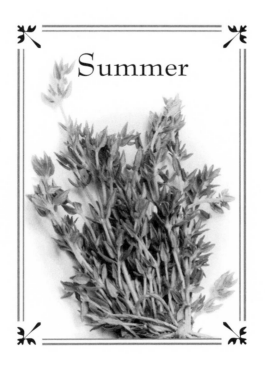

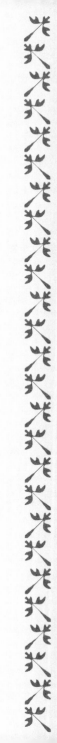

The Summer Months
June, July, August

Summer is the season of the soul that signals manifestation and full expression—the foundation for which is mental clarity, concentration, and focus. Your body, mind, heart, and spirit are energized and motivated, moving your thoughts into action. Fortitude, courage, and confidence help to bring your heart and soul's desire to fruition. Summer is the season that symbolizes the masculine and represents the young-adult stage of your life.

~❧ June ☙~

June is the first Summer month—a time to gain clarity, and to concentrate and focus on what you want to manifest in the world. This lays a strong foundation for achieving your goals. The essential oils for this month are Rosemary for mental clarity, Basil for concentration, Lemon for objectivity, and Peppermint for mental energy.

Rosemary

Best essential oil for mental clarity.

> *Clarity of mind means clarity*
> *of passion, too; this is why a great*
> *and clear mind loves ardently*
> *and sees distinctly what it loves.*
> –Blaise Pascal

LATIN NAME: *Rosmarinus officinalis*

EXTRACTED FROM: Leaves

PSYCHOLOGICAL PROPERTIES: Promotes clear thoughts. Rejuvenates, energizes, and motivates. Dispels apathy and mental fatigue. Relieves nervous exhaustion.

SUBTLE PROPERTIES: Promotes mental clarity. Strengthens and centers the mind. Promotes insights and true understanding. Enhances memory. Associated with the archangel Gabriel in the angelic realm and the kestrel (small falcon) in the animal kingdom.

JUNE 1
Aromatic affirmation with Rosemary

Sit quietly. Close your eyes. Take three slow, relaxed, deep breaths. Open your eyes. Put a drop of Rosemary on a tissue and inhale the aroma through your nose. Pause and inhale again. Say out loud or internally the following affirmation: "My mind is clear and centered. My thoughts are focused and strong."

Rosemary helps to clear, strengthen, and focus your mind.

Aromatic emotional self-discovery with Rosemary

Sit quietly. Close your eyes. Take three slow, relaxed, deep breaths. Open your eyes. Put a drop of Rosemary on a tissue and inhale the aroma through your nose. Pause and inhale again. Ask yourself the following questions and jot down your answers and reflections on a piece of paper.

> ⤙ What does "mental clarity" mean to me?
> ⤙ When have I experienced mental clarity?
> ⤙ In what areas of my life would I like to have more mental clarity?
> ⤙ What supports mental clarity for me?
> ⤙ What interferes with mental clarity for me?
> ⤙ How do I benefit from having mental clarity?

Inhale the aroma of Rosemary again and intend that you are breathing in and experiencing mental clarity. Review your answers to the above questions. Reflect and jot down any additional notes.

Rosemary helps you to experience mental clarity and to understand its role in your life.

JUNE 3
Aromatic clearing ceremony with Rosemary

While standing comfortably with your feet slightly apart, close your eyes. Take three slow, relaxed, deep breaths. Open your eyes. Put a drop of Rosemary on a tissue and inhale the aroma through your nose. Pause and inhale again. With your dominant hand, make three counterclockwise (up on left, down on right) circles in front of your forehead, then your heart, and finally your stomach area, without touching. Then raise your hand in front of your mouth and blow forcefully across your palm with the intention that you are releasing anything that hinders you from having a clear, focused mind.

Rosemary helps to promote mental clarity and focus, and to clear away mental fog and confusion.

JUNE 4
Aromatic blessing with Rosemary

Sit quietly. Close your eyes. Take three slow, relaxed, deep breaths. Open your eyes. Put a drop of Rosemary on a tissue and inhale the aroma through your nose. Pause and inhale again. Say out loud or internally: "Bless me with the gift of mental clarity and strength. Bless me with insights and true understanding. May they guide and direct me to take right action."

Rosemary helps you to experience mental clarity, mental strength, and true understanding.

JUNE 5
Aromatic activity with Rosemary

Sit quietly. Close your eyes. Take three slow, relaxed, deep breaths. Open your eyes. Put a drop of Rosemary on a tissue and inhale the aroma through your nose. Pause and inhale again. Imagine a bright white light coming from the forefinger of your dominant hand. Touch the center of your forehead and intend that it is clearing and illuminating your mind. Touch the center of your chest and intend that it is filling your heart with the clarity and purpose of authentic love. Touch the center of your stomach area and intend that it is strengthening and supporting your actions. Know that you can intentionally touch these places to bring clarity to your thoughts, feelings, and actions.

Rosemary helps to promote and integrate clarity of mind, heart, and will.

JUNE 6
Aromatic visualization with Rosemary

Sit quietly. Close your eyes. Take three slow, relaxed, deep breaths. Open your eyes. Put a drop of Rosemary on a tissue and inhale the aroma through your nose. Pause and inhale again. Visualize a beautiful garden. Walk around and notice all that is here. Notice how clear it is and how easy it is to see the details of each flower and leaf. Sit in a comfortable place. Become aware of the ways in which this garden promotes clarity and understanding of your feelings. Respond to the following sentences and allow yourself to receive the answers—in words, images, thoughts, or feelings.

> I am _____.
> I feel _____.
> I desire _____.
> I will _____.
> I love _____.
> I know _____.
> I learn _____.
> I teach _____.

Rosemary helps to bring you clarity and understanding of your inner world.

Aromatic prayer with Rosemary

Sit quietly. Close your eyes. Take three slow, relaxed, deep breaths. Open your eyes. Put a drop of Rosemary on a tissue and inhale the aroma through your nose. Pause and inhale again. Pray out loud or internally: "Great Spirit, may I clearly feel Your holy presence. May I clearly hear Your sacred words. May I clearly see Your blessed image. May I clearly understand what You intend for me. May my intentions align perfectly with Yours. Amen."

Rosemary helps you to be clear in your intention to serve your highest purpose in alignment with the Divine.

Basil

Best essential oil for concentration.

> *Concentration is my motto—*
> *first honesty, then industry,*
> *then concentration.*
> –Andrew Carnegie

LATIN NAME: *Ocimum basilicum*

EXTRACTED FROM: Flowering plant

PSYCHOLOGICAL PROPERTIES: Encourages and increases concentration. Promotes mental clarity, especially for making choices. Relieves mental fatigue.

SUBTLE PROPERTIES: Increases ability to concentrate. Uplifts and clears the mind. Heightens awareness of all the senses. Associated with the panther in the animal kingdom.

JUNE 8
Aromatic affirmation with Basil

Sit quietly. Close your eyes. Take three slow, relaxed, deep breaths. Open your eyes. Put a drop of Basil on a tissue and inhale the aroma through your nose. Pause and inhale again. Say out loud or internally the following affirmation: "I am able to easily concentrate on what needs and deserves my full attention. My mind is clear, awake, and alert."

Basil helps you to concentrate with a clear, awake, and alert mind.

Aromatic emotional self-discovery with Basil

Sit quietly. Close your eyes. Take three slow, relaxed, deep breaths. Open your eyes. Put a drop of Basil on a tissue and inhale the aroma through your nose. Pause and inhale again. Ask yourself the following questions and jot down your answers and reflections on a piece of paper.

- What does being able to "concentrate" mean to me?
- What helps me to concentrate?
- What interferes with my ability or willingness to concentrate?
- In what areas of my life am I able to concentrate?
- In what areas of my life am I not able to concentrate?
- How does being able to concentrate benefit me?

Inhale the aroma of Basil through your nose again and intend that you are breathing in the ability to concentrate. Review your answers to the above questions. Reflect and jot down any additional notes.

Basil helps you to concentrate and to understand what supports and interferes with your ability to concentrate.

84

DAILY AROMATHERAPY

Aromatic attracting ceremony with Basil

Sit quietly. Close your eyes. Take three slow, relaxed, deep breaths. Open your eyes. Put a drop of Basil on a tissue and inhale the aroma through your nose. Pause and inhale again. Light a candle. As you look at the candle, imagine its radiant light increasing your ability to concentrate. Intend that your mind is cleared and uplifted, and your mental acuity and awareness are heightened. Observe how this affects you on all levels—body, mind, heart, and spirit. Once again, inhale Basil from the tissue and notice your ability to fully concentrate.

Basil helps you to concentrate and heightens your awareness.

Aromatic blessing with Basil

Sit quietly. Close your eyes. Take three slow, relaxed, deep breaths. Open your eyes. Put a drop of Basil on a tissue and inhale the aroma through your nose. Pause and inhale again. Say out loud or internally the following blessing: "Bless all of my senses and how they help me perceive the world. Bless the gift of seeing and the beauty I behold. Bless the gift of hearing and the music I enjoy. Bless the gift of smelling and the aromas I savor. Bless the gift of tasting and the foods I appreciate. Bless the gift of touching and all the ways it nurtures me."

Basil helps to heighten your awareness of all of your senses, and helps you to appreciate them.

Aromatic activity with Basil

Sit quietly. Close your eyes. Take three slow, relaxed, deep breaths. Open your eyes. Put a drop of Basil on a tissue and inhale the aroma through your nose. Pause and inhale again. Choose a piece of food to eat. Choose something you really enjoy. Concentrate on looking at this food—as if seeing it for the first time. Notice its color, texture, and shape. Smell it and reflect upon the aroma. Taste the food and concentrate on the sensation. Be aware of the complexity of the flavor in your mouth and notice what you experience as you swallow. Practice this conscious-eating activity for a few minutes, staying completely focused on experiencing the food. Notice any thoughts and emotions you have as you eat with this level of clarity and attention.

Basil helps you to be more mindful—integrating concentration, mental clarity, and sense awareness.

JUNE 13
Aromatic visualization with Basil

Sit quietly. Close your eyes. Take three slow, relaxed, deep breaths. Open your eyes. Put a drop of Basil on a tissue and inhale the aroma through your nose. Pause and inhale again. Visualize a beautiful garden. Concentrate on experiencing this early-Summer garden with each of your senses. What do you see? What do you hear? What aromas are present? What is the temperature of the air against your skin? What does the sun feel like? Concentrate on being fully present, as much as possible, and notice what it is like for you. From this state of mind, look around and notice if there is anything that needs to be done, such as weeding, watering, or pruning. Observe and determine what this garden needs. Now, in your imagination, tend to this garden. As you do, become aware of how its needs may relate to your own needs. What tending do *you* need? Know that you are able to be fully present and aware of your needs, and can tend to them for your increased sense of well-being.

Basil helps to promote concentration and present awareness, enabling you to notice what is needed in your life.

JUNE 14
Aromatic prayer with Basil

Sit quietly. Close your eyes. Take three slow, relaxed, deep breaths. Open your eyes. Put a drop of Basil on a tissue and inhale the aroma through your nose. Pause and inhale again. Pray out loud or internally: "I give thanks, O Holy One, for the ability to concentrate with a clear mind, heart, and spirit. Help them to work together in me, in harmony, so that I may act with integrity. May I concentrate on growing in Your wisdom. Amen."

Basil helps you to concentrate and have clarity in order to integrate divine wisdom in your mind, heart, and spirit.

Lemon

Best essential oil for objectivity.

> ... *A finely tempered nature longs*
> *to escape from the personal life*
> *into the world of objective*
> *perception and thought.*
> –Albert Einstein

LATIN NAME: *Citrus limonum*

EXTRACTED FROM: Rind

PSYCHOLOGICAL PROPERTIES: Refreshes and energizes. Promotes mental clarity and ability to concentrate. Uplifts and relieves mild depression.

SUBTLE PROPERTIES: Promotes objectivity, mental clarity, and the ability to focus. Clears emotional confusion and misunderstandings. Helps to alleviate fear, especially fear of emotional involvement. Associated with the archangel Uriel in the angelic realm and the giraffe in the animal kingdom.

JUNE 15
Aromatic affirmation with Lemon

Sit quietly. Close your eyes. Take three slow, relaxed, deep breaths. Open your eyes. Put a drop of Lemon on a tissue and inhale the aroma through your nose. Pause and inhale again. Say out loud or internally the following affirmation:

"My mind is clear and objective in ways that are most helpful and for the highest good."

Lemon helps you to experience objectivity through mental clarity.

JUNE 16
Aromatic emotional self-discovery with Lemon

Sit quietly. Close your eyes. Take three slow, relaxed, deep breaths. Open your eyes. Put a drop of Lemon on a tissue and inhale the aroma through your nose. Pause and inhale again. Ask yourself the following questions and jot down your answers and reflections on a piece of paper.

-- What does "objectivity" mean to me?
-- What promotes my ability to be objective?
-- What interferes with my ability to be objective?
-- In what areas of my life is it helpful to be objective?
-- How does being objective benefit me?

Inhale the aroma of Lemon again and intend that you are breathing in the ability to be objective. Review your answers to the above questions. Reflect and jot down any additional notes.

Lemon helps you to be objective in your thinking and to understand the dynamics of objectivity in your life.

JUNE 17
Aromatic integrating ceremony with Lemon

Sit quietly. Close your eyes. Take three slow, relaxed, deep breaths. Open your eyes. Put a drop of Lemon on a tissue and inhale through your nose. Pause and inhale again. Pour some water into a glass. Hold the glass of water with both hands and intend that it is imbued with light and the ability to be objective—an objectivity that clears away emotional confusion and misunderstandings. As you drink the water, think: "I am filled with light. I am able to think clearly and be objective." When you have finished drinking the water, feel and experience being able to think objectively, free of emotional confusion.

Lemon helps you to become objective and mentally clear without cognitive and emotional misunderstandings.

JUNE 18
Aromatic blessing with Lemon

Sit quietly. Close your eyes. Take three slow, relaxed, deep breaths. Open your eyes. Put a drop of Lemon on a tissue and inhale the aroma through your nose. Pause and inhale again. Say out loud or internally the following blessing: "Bless my capacity to observe and understand from a clear and objective perspective. Bless my mind, heart, and spirit as they perceive with detached loving-kindness. Bless the gift of being objective with wisdom and compassion."

Lemon helps you to experience being objective and to understand the blessing of wise and loving objectivity.

Aromatic activity with Lemon

Sit quietly. Close your eyes. Take three slow, relaxed, deep
breaths. Open your eyes. Put a drop of Lemon on a tissue
and inhale the aroma through your nose. Pause and inhale
again. Think of a person or situation that upsets you in some
way. Without judgment, notice how your feelings affect your
thoughts, emotions, opinions, and behaviors. Now inhale
Lemon again, and allow an image to form that represents
that person or situation. Hold your arms out in front of you
and visualize that image in the palms of your hands. Begin
to move your hands. Bring them together and then move
them apart. Turn the image over. Bring the image close to
you and then move it away. Put it in your right hand and then
your left. Notice your thoughts and feelings as you move the
image around. As you observe, discover which position helps
you to experience the most objectivity, without judgment, of
this person or situation. How are you holding it? Are you
moving it or is it still? Notice what it's like for you to experience this objectivity.

Lemon helps you to be objective toward what you observe,
and to understand how this objectivity affects you.

JUNE 20
Aromatic visualization with Lemon

Sit quietly. Close your eyes. Take three slow, relaxed, deep
breaths. Open your eyes. Put a drop of Lemon on a tissue
and inhale the aroma through your nose. Pause and inhale

again. Visualize a beautiful garden. Stand on the periphery of this Summer garden and simply observe for a moment. What do you see? How do you feel? Then, imagine entering this garden for the first time. It is unfamiliar to you and you have no influence here. You cannot change anything. What can you tell about the person who created this place? What can you tell from the plants that were chosen to be here? How is the weather affecting this garden? Are there any animals that have chosen to be here? What can you learn by just observing?

Lemon helps you to be objective in your observations, and to understand that you can learn from being objective.

JUNE 21
Aromatic prayer with Lemon

Sit quietly. Close your eyes. Take three slow, relaxed, deep breaths. Open your eyes. Put a drop of Lemon on a tissue and inhale the aroma through your nose. Pause and inhale again. Pray out loud or internally: "All-Seeing One, You who knows the past, the future, and the fullness of the present. Help me to observe my life objectively and clearly so that my understanding and wisdom deepen. May I be released from attachment to my own 'story' so that I may rest and trust in Your 'story' for me. Amen."

Lemon helps you to be objective so you can be released from attachment to limited human understanding and perspective.

Peppermint

Best essential oil for mental energy.

> *The most powerful factors in*
> *the world are clear ideas in the minds*
> *of energetic men of good will.*
> –J. Arthur Thomson

LATIN NAME: *Mentha piperita*

EXTRACTED FROM: Flowering plant

PSYCHOLOGICAL PROPERTIES: Refreshes, energizes, and uplifts the mind. Relieves mental fatigue.

SUBTLE PROPERTIES: Energizes and refreshes the mind. Promotes mental alertness and clarity. Encourages insightful thinking, especially in discovering one's hidden gifts and strengths. Associated with the bee in the animal kingdom.

JUNE 22
Aromatic affirmation with Peppermint

Sit quietly. Close your eyes. Take three slow, relaxed, deep breaths. Open your eyes. Put a drop of Peppermint on a tissue and inhale the aroma through your nose. Pause and inhale again. Say out loud or internally the following affirmation: "I am awake and alert. My mind is clear and energized."

Peppermint helps to energize the mind and promotes mental clarity and awareness.

Aromatic emotional self-discovery with Peppermint

Sit quietly. Close your eyes. Take three slow, relaxed, deep breaths. Open your eyes. Put a drop of Peppermint on a tissue and inhale the aroma through your nose. Pause and inhale again. Ask yourself the following questions and jot down your answers and reflections on a piece of paper.

- What does "mental energy" mean to me?
- In what area of my life do I experience mental energy?
- In what areas of my life would I like to experience more mental energy?
- What helps my ability to be mentally energetic?
- What hinders my ability to be mentally energetic?
- How does being mentally energetic benefit me?

Inhale the aroma of Peppermint again and feel mentally energetic. Review your answers to the above questions. Reflect and jot down any additional notes.

Peppermint helps you to experience mental energy and to understand its dynamics in your life.

Aromatic manifesting ceremony with Peppermint

Sit quietly. Close your eyes. Take three slow, relaxed, deep breaths. Open your eyes. Find or create an object that represents "mental energy" to you, such as a glowing lamp, a picture of a brilliant scientist, or the image of a lightning bolt. Put a drop of Peppermint on a tissue and inhale the aroma through your nose. Pause and inhale again. Hold your hands over or around the object as you send the intention and quality of mental energy. From now on, whenever you see, touch, or think about this object, your mind will become comfortably energized and refreshed.

Peppermint helps to energize and refresh your mind.

Aromatic blessing with Peppermint

Sit quietly. Close your eyes. Take three slow, relaxed, deep breaths. Open your eyes. Put a drop of Peppermint on a tissue and inhale the aroma through your nose. Pause and inhale again. Say out loud or internally: "Bless my mind and each clear thought that I have. Bless the gift of each insight. Bless my capacity to be alert. Bless the precious treasure of awareness."

Peppermint helps you to be awake and alert, and ever mindful that it is a blessed gift.

Aromatic activity with Peppermint

Sit quietly. Close your eyes. Take three slow, relaxed, deep breaths. Open your eyes. Put a drop of Peppermint on a tissue and inhale the aroma through your nose. Pause and inhale again. Lay your hands, one on top of the other, over your stomach area and say: "May I be aware of and embody 'right action.'" Inhale Peppermint again. Lay your hands, one on top of the other, over your heart area and say: "May I have clarity and insight into my feelings and emotions." Inhale Peppermint again. Hold your hands in front of your forehead, without touching, and say: "May my mind be clear, awake, and alert." Lay your hands over your heart again and say: "I integrate all of this into my being, at this moment."

Peppermint helps to promote strong, clear insights and awareness to assist your thoughts, feelings, and actions.

Aromatic visualization with Peppermint

Sit quietly. Close your eyes. Take three slow, relaxed, deep breaths. Open your eyes. Put a drop of Peppermint on a tissue and inhale the aroma through your nose. Pause and inhale again. Visualize a beautiful garden. Look around and notice all that is in this Summer garden. Be acutely aware of every detail. Notice that it is being well-tended and receiving all that is needed to keep it healthy, thriving, and beautiful—

except for one area. This area is overgrown. Near this over-grown area is a large golden bowl in which a beautiful, clear fire is burning. Next to the bowl is a Peppermint plant. Gently pick a few leaves and place them in the fire. As the scent of Peppermint is released into the air, take a deep and energizing breath. Begin working in the overgrown area, weeding and clipping, until it is just as you want it to be. Now look around this garden with a clear, refreshed vision, appreciating all that is growing and vital here.

Peppermint helps you to feel replenished and energetic, so you can take care of what needs to be done.

JUNE 28
Aromatic prayer with Peppermint

Sit quietly. Close your eyes. Take three slow, relaxed, deep breaths. Open your eyes. Put a drop of Peppermint on a tissue and inhale the aroma through your nose. Pause and inhale again. Pray out loud or internally: "Infinite Mind, clear and energize my human mind so that I may align with Yours. Help me to receive the insights You offer so generously. Help me to be awake and alert to all the ways You are in my life. Amen."

Peppermint helps to clear and energize your mind, increasing your awareness of the Divine and its presence in your life.

End-of-the-Month Days

Write an aromatic affirmation for mental fitness

In a small glass container, mix together:

> 6 drops Rosemary for mental clarity
> 4 drops Basil for concentration
> 2 drops Peppermint for mental energy

Have a pen and paper ready. Sit quietly. Close your eyes. Take three slow, relaxed, deep breaths. Open your eyes. Put a drop of your blend on a tissue and inhale the aroma through your nose. Pause and inhale again. Prepare to write an affirmation for mental fitness. Be clear about your intention. Now write a positive statement about yourself that describes having already achieved that intention in body, mind, heart, and spirit, as if it is already a reality—for example, "My mind is clear, focused, and energized." Allow your affirmation to come sincerely from within. Be as specific as possible. Read it out loud and put it in a place to see throughout the day. Read it often today.

JUNE 30
Aromatic ceremony to honor Summer

Make a blend to honor Summer. In a small glass container, mix together:

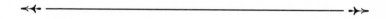

5 drops Rosemary for mental clarity
2 drops Peppermint for mental energy
1 drop Pine for willpower
1 drop Tea Tree for energizing on all levels
3 drops Ginger for manifesting

Gather together in front of you on a table: a large piece of heavy paper such as poster board or cardboard (about eighteen by twelve inches), a yellow crayon or marker, glue, and magazines and/or a variety of colored markers. In the middle of the paper, draw a bright golden sun or create it as a collage with bits of colored paper. Sit quietly. Close your eyes. Take three slow, relaxed, deep breaths. Open your eyes. Put a drop of your Summer blend on a tissue and inhale the aroma through your nose. Pause and inhale again, and as you do, reflect upon the goals in your life that you are currently manifesting or working on manifesting. Write those goals somewhere on the poster board. Now draw a picture or make a collage of an image next to each goal. Inhale your blend once again as you focus on the golden sun in the center of the paper. Draw a golden ray traveling from the center of the sun to each goal and image, and as you do, be aware that the energy of the Summer sun is activating and energizing you as you manifest your desires this season. Place this picture where you can see it, and add goals, images, and golden rays whenever you want.

⤳ July ⤶

July is the second Summer month—a time to exert and demonstrate your energy and willpower to achieve your aspirations, supported by unwavering confidence and courage. The essential oils for this month are Pine for willpower, Cinnamon for self-confidence, Thyme to support the masculine, Tea Tree for energizing on all levels, and German Chamomile for truthful expression.

Pine

Best essential oil for willpower.

> *Lack of willpower*
> *has caused more failure than*
> *lack of intelligence or ability.*
> –Flower A. Newhouse

LATIN NAME: *Pinus sylvestris*

EXTRACTED FROM: Needles

PSYCHOLOGICAL PROPERTIES: Refreshes and uplifts. Eases mental fatigue and mild depression. Relieves anxiety and stress.

SUBTLE PROPERTIES: Restores and builds willpower and self-confidence. Energizes. Associated with the moose in the animal kingdom.

Aromatic affirmation with Pine

Sit quietly. Close your eyes. Take three slow, relaxed, deep breaths. Open your eyes. Put a drop of Pine on a tissue and inhale the aroma through your nose. Pause and inhale again. Say out loud or internally the following affirmation: "My will is strong. I am able to manifest my dreams and goals."

Pine helps you to strengthen and energize your willpower in order to achieve your goals.

Aromatic emotional self-discovery with Pine

Sit quietly. Close your eyes. Take three slow, relaxed, deep breaths. Open your eyes. Put a drop of Pine on a tissue and inhale the aroma through your nose. Pause and inhale again. Ask yourself the following questions and jot down your answers and reflections on a piece of paper.

- What does "willpower" mean to me?
- In what areas of my life do I exert my willpower?
- When I exert my willpower, how do I feel?
- What enhances my willpower?
- What decreases my willpower?
- How do I benefit from having willpower?

Inhale the aroma of Pine again and intend that you are breathing in willpower. Review your answers to the above questions. Reflect and jot down any additional notes.

Pine helps to build your willpower and to understand its dynamics in your life.

Aromatic clearing ceremony with Pine

While standing comfortably with your feet slightly apart, close your eyes. Take three slow, relaxed, deep breaths. Open your eyes. Put a drop of Pine on a tissue and inhale the aroma through your nose. Pause and inhale again. Put the tissue down. With your dominant hand, make three counterclockwise (up on the left, down on the right) circles in front of your forehead, then your heart, and finally your stomach area, without touching. Then raise your hand in front of your mouth and blow forcefully across your palm, with the intention that you are releasing all that prevents you from accessing the power of your will.

Pine helps you to access your personal willpower and to be confident in letting go of all that prevents you from appropriately using it.

Aromatic blessing with Pine

Sit quietly. Close your eyes. Take three slow, relaxed, deep breaths. Open your eyes. Put a drop of Pine on a tissue and inhale the aroma through your nose. Pause and inhale again. Say out loud or internally the following blessing: "Bless my power of will. May it serve me well as I pursue my dreams and purpose. May it assist me in living a happy and good life.

Bless all that I have accomplished and will accomplish through my power of will."

Pine helps you to use your willpower to attain your goals, dreams, and purpose.

JULY 5
Aromatic activity with Pine

Sit quietly. Close your eyes. Take three slow, relaxed, deep breaths. Open your eyes. Put a drop of Pine on a tissue and inhale the aroma through your nose. Pause and inhale again. Think of a time in your life when you used your willpower to pursue and achieve something that you needed or truly wanted. It can be a small thing such as ordering food you really wanted at a restaurant, or a big thing such as being sure you got the recognition you deserved. Now close your eyes and notice how it feels to remember that experience. Bring back the memory of focusing the power of your will on your goal. What do you notice? Pay attention to any sensations in your body, any thoughts, or any emotions. Now, imagine moving your body in such a way that represents this experience of willpower. Open your eyes, inhale Pine again, and this time, actually move your body in the way that you imagined—a way that enhances your willpower. Whenever you desire to activate your willpower, make this movement or just imagine making this movement. Notice how your willpower more quickly and easily becomes available to you.

Pine helps to strengthen and energize your willpower and makes it more accessible to you.

Aromatic visualization with Pine

Sit quietly. Close your eyes. Take three slow, relaxed, deep breaths. Open your eyes. Put a drop of Pine on a tissue and inhale the aroma through your nose. Pause and inhale again. Visualize a beautiful garden. Imagine what this Summer garden would look like if it were designed to represent "willpower." What kind of plants would be there? What colors would the plants be? What characteristics would the plants have? In your mind's eye, make these changes in the garden. You have the influence and ability to shift and change this garden so that it is awe-inspiring. Enjoy creating and experimenting with various changes. Notice how, by simply focusing your will and intention, the needed changes take place. Allow this garden to burst with strength and vitality. Take some time enjoying what you have created and willed into reality.

Pine helps you to access your willpower and to understand how you relate to it.

Aromatic prayer with Pine

Sit quietly. Close your eyes. Take three slow, relaxed, deep breaths. Open your eyes. Put a drop of Pine on a tissue and inhale the aroma through your nose. Pause and inhale again. Pray out loud or internally: "Great Spirit, Creator, You who willed this universe into being, help me to use my personal will in ways that bring me into greater alignment with my

true nature, my highest good, my life purpose, and the ful-
fillment of Your will. May my will become Your instrument.
Amen."

Pine helps you to align your personal will with the divine
will, for the highest good of all.

Cinnamon

Best essential oil for self-confidence.

*Self-confidence is the first requisite
to great undertakings.*
–Samuel Johnson

LATIN NAME: *Cinnamomum verum*

EXTRACTED FROM: Bark or leaf

PSYCHOLOGICAL PROPERTIES: Invigorates. Strengthens.
Relieves mild, lethargic depression.

SUBTLE PROPERTIES: Promotes self-confidence. Strengthens
willpower and courage. Invigorates. Associated with
the raven in the animal kingdom.

JULY 8
Aromatic affirmation with Cinnamon

Sit quietly. Close your eyes. Take three slow, relaxed, deep
breaths. Open your eyes. Put a drop of Cinnamon on a tissue and inhale the aroma through your nose. Pause and
inhale again. Say out loud or internally the following affirmation: "I am confident that I can achieve my goals and
attain my desires. My confidence is natural, appropriate, and
authentic."

Cinnamon helps you to experience genuine self-confidence.

Aromatic emotional self-discovery with Cinnamon

Sit quietly. Close your eyes. Take three slow, relaxed, deep breaths. Open your eyes. Put a drop of Cinnamon on a tissue and inhale the aroma through your nose. Pause and inhale again. Ask yourself the following questions and jot down your answers and reflections on a piece of paper.

- What does "self-confidence" mean to me?
- In what areas of my life am I self-confident?
- In what areas of my life do I lack self-confidence?
- What helps me to feel self-confident?
- What hinders my ability to feel self-confident?
- How would increased self-confidence benefit me?

Inhale the aroma of Cinnamon again and intend that you are breathing in a sense of self-confidence. Review your answers to the above questions. Reflect and jot down any additional notes.

Cinnamon helps you to be self-confident and to understand its dynamics in your life.

JULY 10
Aromatic attracting ceremony with Cinnamon

Sit quietly. Close your eyes. Take three slow, relaxed, deep breaths. Open your eyes. Put a drop of Cinnamon on a tissue and inhale the aroma through your nose. Pause and inhale again. Light a candle. As you look at the candle, experience its radiant light filling you with confidence and courage in your body, mind, heart, and spirit. Inhale Cinnamon once again. Feel strong, confident, and invigorated.

Cinnamon helps you to embody confidence and courage.

JULY 11
Aromatic blessing with Cinnamon

Sit quietly. Close your eyes. Take three slow, relaxed, deep breaths. Open your eyes. Put a drop of Cinnamon on a tissue and inhale the aroma through your nose. Pause and inhale again. Say out loud or internally: "Bless each challenge that I encounter. May I meet it with confidence. Bless each opportunity I have to respond with courage. Bless all the ways in which I am growing into my true, confident self."

Cinnamon helps you to grow in confidence and courage.

JULY 12
Aromatic activity with Cinnamon

While standing comfortably with your feet slightly apart, close your eyes. Take three slow, relaxed, deep breaths. Open your eyes. Put a drop of Cinnamon on a tissue and inhale the aroma through your nose. Pause and inhale again. Bend your knees slightly and relax your shoulders. Take a deep breath, filling your stomach. With the exhalation, make a sound that expresses what you want to express at this moment. The sound might be soft or loud. It might be a note, a word, a shout, a whisper, or a song. It is an expression of you for this moment. Change the sound if you need to. Let the sound fill the area you are in. Notice how you are feeling. Practice until you are confidently "sounding" your True Self.

Cinnamon helps to give you the confidence you need to express your True Self.

Aromatic visualization with Cinnamon

Sit quietly. Close your eyes. Take three slow, relaxed, deep breaths. Open your eyes. Put a drop of Cinnamon on a tissue and inhale the aroma through your nose. Pause and inhale again. Visualize a beautiful garden. Walk into this Summer garden and experience the sun as it bathes you and the garden in warm, golden light. Notice the lushness. Delight in the rich beauty and in your capacity to fully experience it. See the vibrant colors of the flowers and the different shades of green. Hear each delicate sound. Notice the warm smell of the fertile earth and enjoy the many other garden aromas— some strong and some faint. Observe how each plant confidently and perfectly expresses its unique nature, in so many ways. Reflect upon how you are able to do this in your life as well.

Cinnamon helps you to be confident in your unique nature and creative expression.

Aromatic prayer with Cinnamon

Sit quietly. Close your eyes. Take three slow, relaxed, deep breaths. Open your eyes. Put a drop of Cinnamon on a tissue and inhale the aroma through your nose. Pause and inhale again. Pray out loud or internally: "Shining Spirit, Source of All, I am confident in You. May I be confidently in service to You. Teach me to courageously express my true nature and highest purpose. May I grow strong and sure. Amen."

Cinnamon helps you to have appropriate confidence and courage in your service to Spirit.

Thyme

Best essential oil to support the masculine. Embodies the spirit of Summer.

> *How beautiful maleness is,*
> *if it finds its right expression.*
> –D. H. Lawrence

LATIN NAME: *Thymus vulgaris*

EXTRACTED FROM: Whole plant

PSYCHOLOGICAL PROPERTIES: Strengthens. Relieves general fatigue and mild depression.

SUBTLE PROPERTIES: Embodies and supports the masculine. Promotes courage, power, strength, energy, willpower, and confidence. Dispels apathy. Associated with the archangel Michael in the angelic realm and the lion in the animal kingdom.

JULY 15
Aromatic affirmation with Thyme

Sit quietly. Close your eyes. Take three slow, relaxed, deep breaths. Open your eyes. Put a drop of Thyme on a tissue and inhale the aroma through your nose. Pause and inhale again. Say out loud or internally the following affirmation: "I welcome the sacred masculine and all that it symbolizes into my body, mind, heart, and spirit."

Thyme helps you to experience the qualities of the masculine.

Aromatic emotional self-discovery with Thyme

Sit quietly. Close your eyes. Take three slow, relaxed, deep breaths. Open your eyes. Put a drop of Thyme on a tissue and inhale the aroma through your nose. Pause and inhale again. Ask yourself the following questions and jot down your answers and reflections on a piece of paper.

> ⤶ What does "the masculine" mean to me? What are its qualities?
>
> ⤶ How do I experience the masculine in my life?
>
> ⤶ Are there ways in which I embrace the masculine? If so, what are they?
>
> ⤶ Are there ways in which I ignore or negatively judge the masculine? If so, what are they?
>
> ⤶ How does embracing the masculine benefit me?

Inhale the aroma of Thyme again and intend that you are breathing in the qualities of the masculine. Review your answers to the above questions. Reflect and jot down any additional notes.

Thyme helps you to embrace and understand balanced masculine qualities.

Aromatic integrating ceremony with Thyme

Sit quietly. Close your eyes. Take three slow, relaxed, deep breaths. Open your eyes. Put a drop of Thyme on a tissue and inhale the aroma through your nose. Pause and inhale again. Pour some water into a glass. Hold the glass of water with both hands and intend that it is imbued with light and the virtuous qualities of the masculine. As you drink the water, think, "I am filled with light and the qualities of the masculine that are beneficial for me and the good of all." When you have finished drinking, experience those qualities filling your body, mind, heart, and spirit.

Thyme helps you to experience and integrate the gifts of virtuous masculine qualities on all levels.

Aromatic blessing with Thyme

Sit quietly. Close your eyes. Take three slow, relaxed, deep breaths. Open your eyes. Put a drop of Thyme on a tissue and inhale the aroma through your nose. Pause and inhale again. Say out loud or internally the following blessing: "Bless the holy masculine in all of its manifestations. Bless the men and women who embody these virtuous qualities in ways that are healthy and balanced. Bless the ability to take action, have confidence, demonstrate strength, and protect. May the masculine principles of the universe work their blessings in me."

Thyme helps you to experience the sacredness of the masculine.

Aromatic activity with Thyme

While standing comfortably and quietly with your feet slightly apart, close your eyes. Take three slow, relaxed, deep breaths. Open your eyes. Put a drop of Thyme on a tissue and inhale the aroma through your nose. Pause and inhale again. Bring your awareness to your body. Take a few deep, energizing breaths, allowing your body to begin to move as you breathe. Let your body move freely. As you move, experiment with making large gestures—take large steps and make large circles with your arms. Move with purpose, strength, and resolve. Experience being active. Notice how it energizes you. Notice how it affects your breathing. Now, choose a song that you know and like, and sing it as loud as you can. Notice how it feels to be moving and singing in this free-form and active manner.

Thyme helps you to experience being physically active and boldly expressive.

Aromatic visualization with Thyme

Sit quietly. Close your eyes. Take three slow, relaxed, deep breaths. Open your eyes. Put a drop of Thyme on a tissue and inhale the aroma through your nose. Pause and inhale again. Visualize a beautiful garden. As you observe this garden, notice in one area a natural stone formation, covered with moss and surrounded by tall trees. Approach it and discover that this place is dedicated to the masculine. What do you find here? Are there plants? Statues? A picture of something? An animal? What do these things mean to you about your relationship with the masculine? Are there any changes you would like to make? Is there something you would like to remove or add? Take some time and make this area and its surroundings exactly as you would like them to be. Now, honor the virtuous qualities of the masculine that are a part of you, and embody them in a balanced, healthy way.

Thyme helps you to experience the masculine and to honor those aspects of yourself that reflect the masculine.

JULY 21
Aromatic prayer with Thyme

Sit quietly. Close your eyes. Take three slow, relaxed, deep breaths. Open your eyes. Put a drop of Thyme on a tissue and inhale the aroma through your nose. Pause and inhale again. Pray out loud or internally: "Father, I give thanks for all the ways in which You protect, guide, and teach me. I give thanks for Your love, Your steady strength, and for all the ways You encourage me to act with purpose, resolve, love, and integrity. Help me to be fierce when I need to be fierce, and to act when I need to act. Imbue me with loving-kindness so that I might be a true child of Yours. Amen."

Thyme helps you to experience the fathering aspect of the Divine.

Tea Tree

Best essential oil for energizing on all levels.

Energy is eternal delight.
–William Blake

LATIN NAME: *Melaleuca alternifolia*

EXTRACTED FROM: Leaves

PSYCHOLOGICAL PROPERTIES: Uplifts. Energizes. Relieves nervous exhaustion and mild depression.

SUBTLE PROPERTIES: Builds vital, life-giving energy on all levels. Promotes confidence. Associated with the otter in the animal kingdom.

JULY 22
Aromatic affirmation with Tea Tree

Sit quietly. Close your eyes. Take three slow, relaxed, deep breaths. Open your eyes. Put a drop of Tea Tree on a tissue and inhale the aroma through your nose. Pause and inhale again. Say out loud or internally the following affirmation: "I embody and radiate life-giving, vital energy in my body, mind, heart, and spirit."

Tea Tree helps you to generate and radiate vital energy on all levels.

JULY 23
Aromatic emotional self-discovery with Tea Tree

Sit quietly. Close your eyes. Take three slow, relaxed, deep breaths. Open your eyes. Put a drop of Tea Tree on a tissue

DAILY AROMATHERAPY

and inhale the aroma through your nose. Pause and inhale again. Ask yourself the following questions and jot down your answers and reflections on a piece of paper.

- ⇥ What does "vital energy" mean to me?
- ⇥ How do I experience vital energy in my body? Mind? Heart? Spirit?
- ⇥ What impedes my vital energy in each of these areas?
- ⇥ What enhances my vital energy in each of these areas?
- ⇥ How does having vital energy benefit me?

Inhale the aroma of Tea Tree again and intend that you are breathing in pure, life-giving vital energy that affects you on all levels of your being. Review your answers to the above questions. Reflect and jot down any additional notes.

Tea Tree helps you to experience vital energy and to understand its dynamics in your life.

JULY 24
Aromatic manifesting ceremony with Tea Tree

Sit quietly. Close your eyes. Take three slow, relaxed, deep breaths. Open your eyes. Find or create an object that represents "vital energy" for you, such as a piece of sweet fruit, or a picture of the sun or the ocean. Set it in front of you. Put a drop of Tea Tree on a tissue and inhale the aroma through your nose. Pause and inhale again. Hold your hands over or around the object as you send the intention of vital energy into that object. From now on, whenever you see, touch, or remember that object, a sense of vital energy will be with you in body, mind, heart, and spirit. If you choose, place the object in a special place as a reminder.

Tea Tree helps you to experience vital energy on all levels.

Aromatic blessing with Tea Tree

Sit quietly. Close your eyes. Take three slow, relaxed, deep breaths. Open your eyes. Put a drop of Tea Tree on a tissue and inhale the aroma through your nose. Pause and inhale again. Say out loud or internally: "Bless the vital energy that creates and maintains all life. Bless the living force that vibrates in stones and plants, sun and stars, animals and people, and me. Bless all that grows and flourishes. Bless all that expresses the sacredness of vital energy."

Tea Tree helps you to experience the blessing of vital energy that is expressed in many forms in our universe.

Aromatic activity with Tea Tree

Sit quietly. Close your eyes. Take three slow, relaxed, deep breaths. Open your eyes. Put a drop of Tea Tree on a tissue and inhale the aroma through your nose. Pause and inhale again. Stand or sit quietly, and exhale, lowering your shoulders. Now begin and intend to breathe "vital energy" into your body. As you inhale, imagine this life-giving energy coursing through you—into your head and neck, through your shoulders and down your arms. Exhale any fatigue or stress. Inhale the energy again and send it throughout your torso, letting it revitalize and energize all your internal organs. As you exhale, release any toxins—physical, emotional, or mental. Now breathe an energizing breath down into your legs, as you feel the tingling of energy throughout your whole body. As you exhale, be aware that you are exhaling all that keeps you from feeling vitally energized. Take a moment to appreciate this constant cycle of energizing and releasing that enlivens your body at all times. Let yourself experience this vital energy and move your body in a way that expresses it. Is there anything you would like to do with this energy right now? If so, act upon it.

Tea Tree helps you to experience vital energy and how it replenishes you.

JULY 27
Aromatic visualization with Tea Tree

Sit quietly. Close your eyes. Take three slow, relaxed, deep breaths. Open your eyes. Put a drop of Tea Tree on a tissue and inhale the aroma through your nose. Pause and inhale again. Visualize a beautiful garden. Stand in the midst of this Summer garden. Become aware of all of your senses. Experience the vibrancy of the colors, the faint and strong smells, and the sounds. Notice the heat of the sun and the temperature of the air. Sense the fertility and warmth of the earth beneath you. See, feel, hear, smell, and even taste the compelling vital energy as it fills and energizes this place and all of its occupants—including you. Notice how this life-giving energy affects you. Draw in the energy of the sun and earth, as the flowers and plants draw it in. Experience yourself as an energetic, living, and growing part of nature.

Tea Tree helps you to embody the vital energy of nature as it fills your senses and sustains you.

JULY 28
Aromatic prayer with Tea Tree

Sit quietly. Close your eyes. Take three slow, relaxed, deep breaths. Open your eyes. Put a drop of Tea Tree on a tissue and inhale the aroma through your nose. Pause and inhale again. Pray out loud or internally: "God of All Life, fill me with Your vital energy. May I dance with You, sing with You, and play with You. May I be filled to overflowing with Your holy exuberance. All of life praises You, Creator of Energy, Creator of Life. I give thanks. Amen."

Tea Tree helps you to experience and appreciate the precious, divine gift of vital energy.

End-of-the-Month Days

Write an aromatic affirmation for willpower and confidence

In a small glass container, mix together:

> 2 drops Pine for willpower
> 5 drops Cinnamon for confidence
> 5 drops Tea Tree for energizing on all levels

Have a pen and paper ready. Sit quietly. Close your eyes. Take three slow, relaxed, deep breaths. Open your eyes. Put a drop of your blend on a tissue and inhale the aroma through your nose. Pause and inhale again. Prepare to write an affirmation for willpower and confidence. Be clear about your intention. Now write a positive statement about yourself that describes having already achieved that intention in body, mind, heart, and spirit, as if it is already a reality—for example, "My willpower is strong and I am confident." Allow your affirmation to come sincerely from within. Be as specific as possible. Read it out loud and put it in a place to see throughout the day. Read it often today.

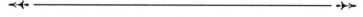

JULY 30
New Summer essential oil: German Chamomile

German Chamomile

Best essential oil for truthful expression.

> *In a time of universal deceit,*
> *telling the truth is a revolutionary act.*
> –George Orwell

LATIN NAME: *Matricaria chamomilla*

EXTRACTED FROM: Blossoms

PSYCHOLOGICAL PROPERTIES: Calms and relaxes. Relieves mild
   depression, anxiety and stress.

SUBTLE PROPERTIES: Supports calm, truthful expression and
   communication. Helps to calm and balance the
   emotions.

Aromatic visualization exercise with German Chamomile

Sit quietly. Close your eyes. Take three slow, relaxed, deep
breaths. Open your eyes. Put a drop of German Chamomile
on a tissue and inhale the aroma through your nose. Pause
and inhale again. Visualize a beautiful, long hallway. On the
walls, mirrors are hung of different shapes, sizes, and styles.
Imagine that each of these mirrors is an expression of you.
They reflect truths that your Higher Self knows and will

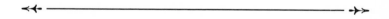

reveal to you now. The truth of a relationship might be shown or truths related to emotions, thoughts, beliefs, family, childhood, or work. Inhale German Chamomile once again. Discover an aspect or experience of your life that you would like to look at more fully, deeply, and truthfully. Allow a question to form and invite its truth to be expressed to you now. Let that question guide you to one of the mirrors. Now watch and discover the truth that is ready to be revealed to you in this moment. Inhale German Chamomile again, and know that this truth will continue to integrate in your body, mind, heart, and spirit in times to come.

German Chamomile helps to support the calm discovery and expression of the truth.

JULY 31
Aromatic activity to energize the home

Sit quietly. Close your eyes. Take three slow, relaxed, deep breaths. Open your eyes. Put a drop of Tea Tree on a tissue and inhale the aroma through your nose. Pause and inhale again. Gather from your garden a bouquet of yellow, red, and orange flowers. If you do not have a garden, purchase a bouquet of flowers with these colors. Sunflowers are especially wonderful. Put these flowers in vases of water and place them throughout your home. These flowers and their colors honor the sun and bring its vibrant energy, the greatest during the Summer, into your home.

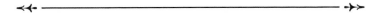

❧ August ❧

August is the last Summer month—a time for the manifestation and achievement of your dreams and desires through personal motivation, passion, and perseverance. The essential oils for this month are Clove for motivation, Ginger for manifesting, Ylang Ylang for passion and enthusiasm, and Fennel for perseverance.

Clove

Best essential oil for motivation.

> *The only lifelong, reliable motivations*
> *are those that come from within,*
> *and one of the strongest of those is*
> *the joy and pride that grow*
> *from knowing that you've just done*
> *something as well as you can do it.*
> –Lloyd Dobens and Clare Crawford-Mason

LATIN NAME: *Eugenia caryophyllata*

EXTRACTED FROM: Buds

PSYCHOLOGICAL PROPERTIES: Uplifts. Strengthens the memory. Revives a tired mind.

SUBTLE PROPERTIES: Motivates on all levels—body, mind, heart, and spirit. Encourages action and promotes achievement. Associated with the fox in the animal kingdom.

AUGUST 1

Aromatic affirmation with Clove

Sit quietly. Close your eyes. Take three slow, relaxed, deep breaths. Open your eyes. Put a drop of Clove on a tissue and inhale the aroma through your nose. Pause and inhale again. Say out loud or internally the following affirmation: "I feel the call to action, in my body. I hear the call to action, in my heart. I know the call to action, in my mind. I respond to the call to action, in spirit."

Clove helps to motivate you to action on all levels.

AUGUST 2

Aromatic emotional self-discovery with Clove

Sit quietly. Close your eyes. Take three slow, relaxed, deep breaths. Open your eyes. Put a drop of Clove on a tissue and inhale the aroma through your nose. Pause and inhale again. Ask yourself the following questions and jot down your answers and reflections on a piece of paper.

- What does "being motivated" mean to me?
- What motivates me?
- In what areas of my life do I need and/or want to be motivated?
- What makes being motivated easier for me?
- What impedes my motivation?
- What are the benefits of being motivated for me?

Inhale the aroma of Clove again and intend that you are breathing in a sense of motivation. Review your answers to the above questions. Reflect and jot down any additional notes.

Clove helps you to experience and understand the dynamics of motivation in your life.

Aromatic clearing ceremony with Clove

While standing comfortably with your feet slightly apart, close your eyes. Take three slow, relaxed, deep breaths. Open your eyes. Put a drop of Clove on a tissue and inhale the aroma through your nose. Pause and inhale again. With your dominant hand, make three counterclockwise (up on the left, down on the right) circles in front of your forehead, then your heart, and lastly, your stomach area, without touching. Raise your hand in front of your mouth and blow forcefully across your palm with the intention that you are releasing all the things that prevent you from being motivated. Inhale Clove again. Embrace the feeling of motivation—the drive, the impulse, the zeal.

Clove helps you to experience motivation and release all that hinders it for you.

Aromatic blessing with Clove

Sit quietly. Close your eyes. Take three slow, relaxed, deep breaths. Open your eyes. Put a drop of Clove on a tissue and inhale the aroma through your nose. Pause and inhale again.

Say out loud or internally the following blessing: "Bless all that motivates me to act and achieve. Bless all that I am motivated to accomplish. Bless each step on this journey that I may walk with integrity, vitality, and authenticity."

Clove helps you to experience motivation and to understand its blessings.

AUGUST 5
Aromatic activity with Clove

While standing comfortably with your feet slightly apart, close your eyes. Take three slow, relaxed, deep breaths. Open your eyes. Put a drop of Clove on a tissue and inhale the aroma through your nose. Pause and inhale again. Think of someone you respect who is currently motivated to achieve something they deeply desire. It may be someone you know personally or someone you know about, such as an artist, athlete, or scientist. Imagine that you can "step into their shoes" and experience their motivation. Move your feet as if you were stepping into those shoes. Now, let yourself fully connect with the feeling of being motivated—with all of your senses. Does it feel right for you? If not, make whatever adjustments you need to, in order to have this sense of motivation fit *you*. Then step out of their shoes. As you do, bring the feeling and experience of being motivated with you. Inhale the aroma of Clove again. Take four steps forward and with each step say, "I am motivated." On the first step, allow this affirmation to fill your feet and legs. On the second step, allow it to move through your stomach area and back. On your third step, allow it to fill your chest, heart, and shoulders, and flow down your arms into your hands. With the final and fourth step, allow it to fill your mind. Say, one more time, "I am motivated." Sense it in every cell of your body. Know that from now on, whenever you want to find your motivation, you can inhale Clove, state the affirmation, and take a step forward.

Clove helps you to experience motivation and notice how it empowers you.

Aromatic visualization with Clove

Sit quietly. Close your eyes. Take three slow, relaxed, deep breaths. Open your eyes. Put a drop of Clove on a tissue and inhale the aroma through your nose. Pause and inhale again. Visualize a beautiful garden. Begin to stroll in this Summer garden. Notice a flash of light near the ground in a bed of flowers. Approach the light and discover it is a mirror, slightly hidden. Pick up the mirror, and look into it. See your future self—the self who has achieved what you hope to achieve. See this future self in great detail. Where do you live? Who is around you? How are you spending your time? How is your health? This future self serves as an internal guide to motivate and coach you, now, to achieve what is important to you in the future. Ask how you can accomplish these goals. Ask for any help or inspiration you might need. Spend a few moments in conversation with this wise aspect of yourself. When you are ready to say goodbye, know that this mirror will continue to be here in the garden, and you can come here to consult with your future self whenever you want or need support for motivation.

Clove helps you to experience motivation by accessing your inner resources so you can achieve your desires.

AUGUST 7
Aromatic prayer with Clove

Sit quietly. Close your eyes. Take three slow, relaxed, deep breaths. Open your eyes. Put a drop of Clove on a tissue and inhale the aroma through your nose. Pause and inhale again. Pray out loud or internally: "Great Motivator who calls forth the universe and all its inhabitants, help me to be all that You desire me to be. Assist me in achieving all that You ask of me. Help me to hear and respond to Your call. May I know deeply that the truest call is the call to You and the greatest achievement is service to You. Amen."

Clove helps to motivate you to respond and surrender to the Divine.

Ginger

Best essential oil for manifesting.

The thought manifests as the word;
The word manifests as the deed;
The deed develops into habit;
And habit hardens into character.
So watch the thought and its ways
with care, And let it spring
from love born out of concern
for all beings.
–The Buddha

LATIN NAME: *Zingiber officinale*

EXTRACTED FROM: Root

PSYCHOLOGICAL PROPERTIES: Revives and uplifts. Warms the emotions.

SUBTLE PROPERTIES: Promotes and supports the manifestation of your heart and soul's desire. Strengthens the will. Attracts prosperity. Promotes courage and confidence. Associated with the archangel Ariel in the angelic realm and the lynx in the animal kingdom.

AUGUST 8
Aromatic affirmation with Ginger

Sit quietly. Close your eyes. Take three slow, relaxed, deep breaths. Open your eyes. Put a drop of Ginger on a tissue and inhale the aroma through your nose. Pause and inhale again. Say out loud or internally the following affirmation: "I manifest all that I desire with confidence, courage, and ease."

Ginger helps you to claim your capacity to manifest.

AUGUST 9
Aromatic emotional self-discovery with Ginger

Sit quietly. Close your eyes. Take three slow, relaxed, deep breaths. Open your eyes. Put a drop of Ginger on a tissue. Inhale the aroma through your nose. Pause and inhale again. Ask yourself the following questions and jot down your answers and reflections on a piece of paper.

- What does "manifesting" mean to me?
- What have I successfully manifested in my life that I truly desired?
- What have I been unable or unwilling to manifest that I truly desire?
- What strengthens my capacity to manifest?
- What interferes with my capacity to manifest?
- How does being able to manifest my desires benefit me?

Inhale the aroma of Ginger again and intend that you are breathing in the ability to manifest your heart and soul's desires. Review your answers to the above questions. Reflect and jot down any additional notes.

Ginger helps you to experience and understand the ability to manifest what you want in your life.

AUGUST 10
Aromatic attracting ceremony with Ginger

Sit quietly. Close your eyes. Take three slow, relaxed, deep breaths. Open your eyes. Put a drop of Ginger on a tissue and inhale through your nose. Pause and inhale again. Light a candle. Experience the radiant light of this candle filling you with the strength and courage to manifest your desires on all levels—body, mind, heart, and spirit. Once again, inhale Ginger from the tissue. Feel yourself filled with the ability to manifest all that you need and want.

Ginger helps you to embody the qualities necessary to manifest what you need and want in your life.

AUGUST 11
Aromatic blessing with Ginger

Sit quietly. Close your eyes. Take three slow, relaxed, deep breaths. Open your eyes. Put a drop of Ginger on a tissue and inhale the aroma through your nose. Pause and inhale again. Say out loud or internally: "Bless my ability to manifest the life I desire. Bless the source of the energy I harness to manifest these dreams. Bless all that manifests through me."

Ginger helps you to experience the process and blessing of manifesting your desires.

AUGUST 12
Aromatic activity with Ginger

Sit quietly. Close your eyes. Take three slow, relaxed, deep breaths. Open your eyes. Put a drop of Ginger on a tissue and inhale the aroma through your nose. Pause and inhale again. On a piece of paper, make a list of twelve things that you would like to manifest in your life. Include accomplishments that you consider large and small, as well as easy and challenging. Now choose one that you are ready to commit to doing or to begin doing today. Circle it on this piece of paper. Take a second piece of paper and write this circled item at the top. List the steps that will be necessary for you to manifest the desired outcome. These may include things you will need to do, as well as emotional adjustments you may need to make. Put these steps in order so that, to the best of your ability, you can see the process of what needs to be done. Inhale Ginger once more from your tissue and think about the first step on the list. Decide the time frame in which you will do this. When you have accomplished it, find a way to celebrate this as a step you have taken toward manifesting a desired goal. Know that each small success enhances your ability to manifest. Then, move on to the next step. Use Ginger to assist you every step of the way. When you have completed this goal, return to your first list, choose another item, and repeat the process.

Ginger helps you to experience the ability to manifest and to take the steps that are needed to accomplish your dreams and goals.

AUGUST 13
Aromatic visualization with Ginger

Sit quietly. Close your eyes. Take three slow, relaxed, deep breaths. Open your eyes. Put a drop of Ginger on a tissue and inhale the aroma through your nose. Pause and inhale again. Visualize a beautiful garden. Find yourself standing in the midst of this Summer garden. Become fully aware that *you,* and your conscious and unconscious creativity, have manifested every exquisite aspect of this garden. You created and manifested the design, the appearance of every plant, the wide array of colors, the beautiful sounds, the exquisite aromas, the temperature, and all the features throughout. Everything here is a reflection of your capacity to manifest what you desire. Be here in this garden, fully present, and aware of all your senses. Remember that you can change whatever you want to change in order to make it a perfect representation of your desires. Enjoy.

Ginger helps you to experience your capacity to creatively manifest your desires.

AUGUST 14
Aromatic prayer with Ginger

Sit quietly. Close your eyes. Take three slow, relaxed, deep breaths. Open your eyes. Put a drop of Ginger on a tissue and inhale the aroma through your nose. Pause and inhale again. Pray out loud or internally: "Great Creator, You who manifested this sacred universe, may all that I manifest be in alignment with, and in service to, Your divine plan. Amen."

Ginger helps you to manifest your desires in alignment with the Creator.

Ylang Ylang

Best essential oil for passion and enthusiasm.

> *Only passions, great passions,*
> *can elevate the soul to great things.*
> –Denis Diderot

LATIN NAME: *Cananga odorata*

EXTRACTED FROM: Flower

PSYCHOLOGICAL PROPERTIES: Promotes a sense of well-being and happiness. Uplifts and relaxes. Relieves stress and tension.

SUBTLE PROPERTIES: Promotes passion and enthusiasm. Encourages confidence and sensuality. Associated with the porpoise in the animal kingdom.

AUGUST 15
Aromatic affirmation with Ylang Ylang

Sit quietly. Close your eyes. Take three slow, relaxed, deep breaths. Open your eyes. Put a drop of Ylang Ylang on a tissue and inhale the aroma through your nose. Pause and inhale again. Say out loud or internally the following affirmation: "I am a passionate and enthusiastic being, radiant with life."

Ylang Ylang helps you to experience your passionate and enthusiastic nature.

Aromatic emotional self-discovery with Ylang Ylang

Sit quietly. Close your eyes. Take three slow, relaxed, deep breaths. Open your eyes. Put a drop of Ylang Ylang on a tissue and inhale the aroma through your nose. Pause and inhale again. Ask yourself the following questions and jot down your answers and reflections on a piece of paper.

> ⤙ What does "enthusiasm" mean to me?
>
> ⤙ How do I experience enthusiasm in my life?
>
> ⤙ What helps me to be enthusiastic?
>
> ⤙ What hinders me from being enthusiastic?
>
> ⤙ How do I express enthusiasm in my life?
>
> ⤙ How is being enthusiastic beneficial for me?

Inhale the aroma of Ylang Ylang again and intend that you are breathing in authentic enthusiasm. Review your answers to the above questions. Reflect and jot down any additional notes.

Ylang Ylang helps you to experience enthusiasm and to understand its dynamics in your life.

AUGUST 17
Aromatic integrating ceremony with Ylang Ylang

Sit quietly. Close your eyes. Take three slow, relaxed, deep breaths. Open your eyes. Put a drop of Ylang Ylang on a tissue and inhale through your nose. Pause and inhale again. Pour some water into a glass. Hold the glass of water with both hands and intend that it is imbued with light and life-affirming passion and enthusiasm. As you drink the water, imagine: "I am filled with light and a great passion for living." When you have finished drinking, experience the sensation of being energized with passion and enthusiasm.

Ylang Ylang helps you to experience and embody passion and enthusiasm.

Aromatic blessing with Ylang Ylang

Sit quietly. Close your eyes. Take three slow, relaxed, deep breaths. Open your eyes. Put a drop of Ylang Ylang on a tissue and inhale the aroma through your nose. Pause and inhale again. Say out loud or internally: "Bless the passion and enthusiasm that bring forth life and vitality. Bless the passion and enthusiasm that create and celebrate. Bless the manifestations of passion and enthusiasm in all their glorious diversity."

Ylang Ylang helps you to experience and fully appreciate the life-affirming qualities of passionate living.

AUGUST 19
Aromatic activity with Ylang Ylang

Sit quietly. Close your eyes. Take three slow, relaxed, deep breaths. Open your eyes. Put a drop of Ylang Ylang on a tissue and inhale the aroma through your nose. Pause and inhale again. Select and listen to a piece of music that moves you in a passionate way. It may be passionately joyful, energizing, romantic, angry, or sad. Notice the specific form of passion that speaks to you. As the music fills your body, allow yourself to move and/or dance to the melody. Pay attention to how you feel. Do you feel invigorated? Do you feel uncomfortable? Allow your body to move freely and experiment. Continue to move and listen to the music until the song is over. Notice how you are feeling at every level—body, mind, heart, and spirit. Has anything changed from how you were feeling before listening to and moving with the music?

Ylang Ylang helps you to experience and experiment with expressing passion through movement and/or dance.

AUGUST 20
Aromatic visualization with Ylang Ylang

Sit quietly. Close your eyes. Take three slow, relaxed, deep breaths. Open your eyes. Put a drop of Ylang Ylang on a tissue and inhale the aroma through your nose. Pause and inhale again. Visualize a beautiful garden. Be aware that this Summer garden is filled with the passionate and enthusiastic energy of nature. Explore and notice the colors, shapes, scents, and sounds that express this passionate energy. Spend some time here. What catches your attention? Be aware if you become more passionate about any particular aspect. In what way does this garden touch, encourage, or express your own passionate and enthusiastic nature?

Ylang Ylang helps you to experience and identify passion and its individual expressions in your life.

AUGUST 21
Aromatic prayer with Ylang Ylang

Sit quietly. Close your eyes. Take three slow, relaxed, deep breaths. Open your eyes. Put a drop of Ylang Ylang on a tissue and inhale the aroma through your nose. Pause and inhale again. Pray out loud or internally: "Beloved God, may I love You above all else. May I long for You above all else. May I see only You. Amen."

Ylang Ylang helps to support your passionate yearning for the Divine.

Fennel

Best essential oil for perseverance.

> *Press on: nothing in the world*
> *can take the place of perseverance.*
> *Talent will not; nothing is more*
> *common than unsuccessful men*
> *with talent. Genius will not;*
> *unrewarded genius is almost*
> *a proverb. Education will not;*
> *the world is full of educated derelicts.*
> *Persistence and determination*
> *alone are omnipotent.*
>
> –Calvin Coolidge

LATIN NAME: *Foeniculum vulgare dulce*

EXTRACTED FROM: Seeds

PSYCHOLOGICAL PROPERTIES: Emotionally fortifies.

SUBTLE PROPERTIES: Promotes perseverance. Encourages
   assertiveness. Motivates and builds confidence,
   especially in communication. Associated with the
   salmon in the animal kingdom.

AUGUST 22
Aromatic affirmation with Fennel

Sit quietly. Close your eyes. Take three slow, relaxed, deep
breaths. Open your eyes. Put a drop of Fennel on a tissue
and inhale the aroma through your nose. Pause and inhale
again. Say out loud or internally the following affirmation:
"I am empowered to persevere as I pursue my goals."

Fennel helps to support your ability to persevere in the pursuit of your goals.

AUGUST 23
Aromatic emotional self-discovery with Fennel

Sit quietly. Close your eyes. Take three slow, relaxed, deep breaths. Open your eyes. Put a drop of Fennel on a tissue and inhale the aroma through your nose. Pause and inhale again. Ask yourself the following questions and jot down your answers and reflections on a piece of paper.

- What does being able to "persevere" mean to me?
- In what areas of my life is it easy for me to persevere?
- In what areas of my life is it challenging for me to persevere?
- What supports and enhances my ability to persevere?
- What interferes with my ability to persevere?
- How does being able to persevere benefit me?

Inhale the aroma of Fennel again and intend that you are breathing in the ability to persevere. Review your answers to the above questions. Reflect and jot down any additional notes.

Fennel helps you to experience and determine the areas of your life that require perseverance.

Aromatic manifesting ceremony with Fennel

Sit quietly. Close your eyes. Take three slow, relaxed, deep breaths. Open your eyes. Find or create an object that represents "perseverance" for you, such as a copy of a diploma or a picture of an accomplished athlete. Set it in front of you. Put a drop of Fennel on a tissue and inhale through your nose. Pause and inhale again. Hold your hands over or around the object as you send the intention of perseverance into that object. From now on, whenever you see, touch, or remember that object, the sense of perseverance will be with you in body, mind, heart, and spirit. If you choose, place the object in a special place as a reminder.

Fennel helps you to experience the ability to persevere, supported by the assertiveness and confidence necessary to achieve your goals.

Aromatic blessing with Fennel

Sit quietly. Close your eyes. Take three slow, relaxed, deep breaths. Open your eyes. Put a drop of Fennel on a tissue and inhale the aroma through your nose. Pause and inhale again. Say out loud or internally the following blessing: "Bless the ability of life to persevere and flourish. Bless all that endures. Bless the part of me that faces challenges yet

DAILY AROMATHERAPY

perseveres. Bless the life force that keeps me growing, expanding, and creating."

Fennel helps you to persevere and endure through challenges large and small in order to reach your goals.

Aromatic activity with Fennel

Sit quietly. Close your eyes. Take three slow, relaxed, deep breaths. Open your eyes. Put a drop of Fennel on a tissue and inhale the aroma through your nose. Pause and inhale again. Reflect on the animal kingdom and the amazing challenges that so many animals experience in living and surviving. Choose an animal that embodies the capacity to persevere for you. Did you choose the emperor penguin, which faces daunting cold in the Antarctic environment, or the salmon that swim so intently upstream? Did you think of the raccoon, which has found extraordinary ways to acclimate to a changing environment? Take a few moments to reflect on your animal and the qualities of perseverance that it demonstrates. Notice other qualities of that animal. Now, imagine that you could become that animal. Shift your body into a position that mimics this animal's stance and move around. Imagine yourself as this animal in a situation that reflects this animal's particular gift for perseverance. Is there a sound, movement, feeling, or other expression that can accompany this? Discover if there is a way in which this animal's gift for perseverance is in any way similar to your own. Perhaps this animal has something to teach you that will help you to persevere. Enjoy "being" this animal for as long as you like.

Fennel helps you to experience, appreciate, and learn perseverance as it is demonstrated by animals in nature.

AUGUST 27
Aromatic visualization with Fennel

Sit quietly. Close your eyes. Take three slow, relaxed, deep breaths. Open your eyes. Put a drop of Fennel on a tissue and inhale the aroma through your nose. Pause and inhale again. Visualize a beautiful garden. As you look around, imagine, in great detail, what this garden might have looked like five to ten years ago. Now imagine what it might look like five to ten years into the future. What is no longer there? What remains? As you imagine what is gone, how do you feel? Why is it gone? As you notice what remains, how do you feel? Why has it persevered? What is the relationship between what is gone and what has persevered?

Fennel helps you to experience perseverance as it pertains to what is transient and what persists.

AUGUST 28
Aromatic prayer with Fennel

Sit quietly. Close your eyes. Take three slow, relaxed, deep breaths. Open your eyes. Put a drop of Fennel on a tissue and inhale the aroma through your nose. Pause and inhale again. Pray out loud or internally: "Great Spirit, help me to persevere in Your service. Teach me how to persevere and to be assertive, when necessary. Help me to know when to persevere and when to let go. May all that I commit to accomplishing be for the highest good and be in accordance with Your purpose. Amen."

Fennel helps you to experience perseverance in accordance with divine guidance as you journey through life.

End-of-the-Month Days

AUGUST 29

Write an aromatic affirmation for manifesting

In a small glass container, mix together:

> 2 drops Clove for motivation
> 1 drop Ginger for manifesting
> 8 drops Ylang Ylang for passion and
> enthusiasm
> 1 drop Fennel for perseverance

Have a pen and paper ready. Sit quietly. Close your eyes. Take three slow, relaxed, deep breaths. Open your eyes. Put a drop of your blend on a tissue and inhale the aroma through your nose. Pause and inhale again. Prepare to write an affirmation for manifesting what you desire. Identify what it is that you intend to manifest. Now write a positive statement about yourself that describes having already achieved that intention in body, mind, heart, and spirit, as if it is already a reality—for example, "I have a wonderful home." Allow your affirmation to come sincerely from within. Be as specific as possible. Read it out loud and put it in a place to see throughout the day. Read it often today.

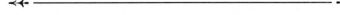

AUGUST 30
Aromatic activity for manifesting

Gather together: an attractive box with a lid that closes, tape, pen or pencil, and pieces of paper. Sit quietly. Close your eyes. Take three slow, relaxed, deep breaths. Open your eyes. Put a drop of Ginger on a tissue and inhale the aroma through your nose. Pause and inhale again. Take a moment to appreciate this box and its beauty. Now write on a piece of paper, "Everything in this box is true." Tape it on the inside of the lid. Inhale Ginger one more time and hold this box for a moment, intending that this "manifesting box" contains and enhances the mental and emotional processes of intentional manifesting. When you are ready, write what you want to manifest in your life on slips of paper—one item per piece of paper. Write your statement in positive terms, as if it is already happening. The statements might be general, such as, "I am financially secure," or more specific, such as, "I pay my bills easily and place money in my savings account every month." As you place each piece of paper into the box, state your intention out loud. When complete, close the lid, inhale Ginger once again, and hold the box, stating in a firm voice, "Everything in this box is true." Now place this box where you can see it and know that all that you desire is manifesting now in your consciousness and in your life.

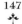

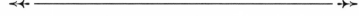

AUGUST 31

Aromatic ceremony to honor your accomplishments this Summer

Choose one of your favorite Summer essential oils: Rosemary, Basil, Lemon, Peppermint, Pine, Cinnamon, Thyme, Tea Tree, German Chamomile, Clove, Ginger, Ylang Ylang, or Fennel. Sit quietly. Close your eyes. Take three slow, relaxed, deep breaths. Open your eyes. Put a drop of your chosen oil on a tissue and inhale the aroma through your nose. Pause and inhale again. Reflect back upon the past Summer season and identify your accomplishments. Don't be modest. Notice each and every goal you have accomplished, from small to large. Inhale your oil once again, and take a large step forward. As you do, say out loud or internally, "I have accomplished _____ this Summer." Inhale your oil again, and take another step, saying out loud or internally, "I have also accomplished _____ in these last few months." With one more step and one final inhalation, say out loud or internally, "I want to be sure I acknowledge accomplishing _____." Now turn around and visualize looking back at yourself prior to taking these three steps. Notice how, in only a few minutes, something has changed within you simply through the process of acknowledging what you have accomplished. Now ask yourself what you might like to do to celebrate what you have accomplished. This could be

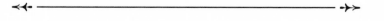

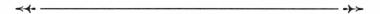

going to a concert, taking a sky-diving lesson, or starting an exercise class. Think of something that would please you and make a commitment to do this for yourself now, to honor your accomplishments this Summer.

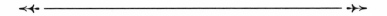

Autumn

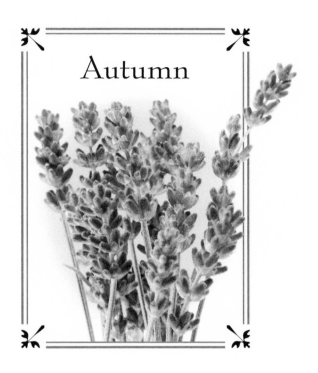

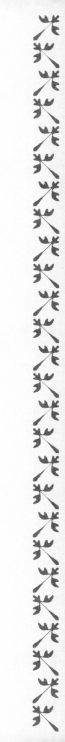

The Autumn Months
September, October, November

Autumn is the season of the soul that signals a time to reflect on your life and assess the health and well-being of your body, mind, heart, and spirit. It is a time for insights and using good judgment regarding your relationships, how you take care of yourself, how you spend your time, and what you have accomplished. Forgiving and accepting your shortcomings, as well as the shortcomings of others, help you pave the way to a peaceful heart. It is also a time to acknowledge and be grateful for the many blessings in your life, and to be generous of spirit. In all of this, healing takes place. Autumn represents the mid-life stage of your life.

⤳ September ⤝

September is the first Autumn month—a time for self-reflection and understanding, the use of good judgment, and the development of insight, awareness, and intuition. The essential oils for this month are Spruce for self-reflection, Fir for self-understanding, Bay Laurel for using good judgment, and Clary Sage for intuition.

Spruce

Best essential oil for self-reflection.

> *By three methods we may learn*
> *wisdom: First, by reflection,*
> *which is noblest; second, by imitation,*
> *which is easiest; and third by*
> *experience, which is the bitterest.*
> –Confucius

LATIN NAME: *Picea mariana*

EXTRACTED FROM: Needles

PSYCHOLOGICAL PROPERTIES: Uplifts. Eases mild depression. Relieves mental exhaustion. Eases stress, anxiety, and tension.

SUBTLE PROPERTIES: Promotes self-reflection with objectivity. Clears the mind for the development of intuition. Associated with the wolf in the animal kingdom.

SEPTEMBER 1
Aromatic affirmation with Spruce

Sit quietly. Close your eyes. Take three slow, relaxed, deep breaths. Open your eyes. Put a drop of Spruce on a tissue and inhale the aroma through your nose. Pause and inhale again. Say out loud or internally the following affirmation: "I can objectively reflect on *who* I am, in both my inner world and the outer world."

Spruce helps you to know yourself through objective self-reflection.

SEPTEMBER 2

Aromatic emotional self-discovery with Spruce

Sit quietly. Close your eyes. Take three slow, relaxed, deep breaths. Open your eyes. Put a drop of Spruce on a tissue and inhale the aroma through your nose. Pause and inhale again. Ask yourself the following questions and jot down your answers and reflections on a piece of paper.

- What does "self-reflection" mean to me?
- What areas of my life support and encourage self-reflection?
- What self-reflection practices work best for me? (Examples are journaling, writing poetry, free-style drawing, or communicating with a friend.)
- What have I learned about myself through self-reflection?
- How do I benefit from self-reflection?

Inhale the aroma of Spruce again and intend that you are breathing in the ability to reflect on who you are. Review your answers to the above questions. Reflect and jot down any additional notes.

Spruce helps you to experience and understand the dynamics of self-reflection in your life.

Aromatic clearing ceremony with Spruce

While standing comfortably with your feet slightly apart, close your eyes. Take three slow, relaxed, deep breaths. Open your eyes. Put a drop of Spruce on a tissue and inhale the aroma through your nose. Pause and inhale again. With your dominant hand, make three counterclockwise (up on the left, down on the right) circles, in front of your forehead, then your heart, and lastly, your stomach area, without touching. Raise your hand in front of your mouth and blow forcefully across your palm with the intention that you are releasing anything that interferes with your capacity and willingness to reflect, objectively, on who you are in the world. Inhale Spruce again and take a few moments to self-reflect.

Spruce helps you to be able to objectively reflect upon who you are in the world and to release the obstacles that hinder the self-reflection process.

Aromatic blessing with Spruce

Sit quietly. Close your eyes. Take three slow, relaxed, deep breaths. Open your eyes. Put a drop of Spruce on a tissue and inhale the aroma through your nose. Pause and inhale again. Say out loud or internally: "Bless all that encourages me to reflect on who I am. Bless the moments in which I look deeply into my heart and soul. Bless all that I learn and all that results from this contemplation. May I grow in wisdom."

Spruce helps you to reflect on who you are, and to understand the blessings of the process.

Aromatic activity with Spruce

Sit or stand quietly. Close your eyes. Take three slow, relaxed, deep breaths. Open your eyes. Put a drop of Spruce on a tissue and inhale the aroma through your nose. Pause and inhale again. Look into a mirror and observe your reflection. Write down what you see and any thoughts and feelings that are present. What is the first perception that comes to you? Is it loving? Critical? Judgmental? Simply notice and name this first response. Then, begin to experiment with other perceptions. If you experienced your reflection lovingly, what would change if you reflected upon your mirror image critically or judgmentally? Notice how different perceptions feel to you. Are they familiar? Unfamiliar? Comfortable? Uncomfortable? Discover if the various perceptions bring your attention to different aspects of yourself such as your physical appearance, your attitude, or your soul. Are some reflections more useful, productive, or enlightening than others? Is there a perception that is most pleasing to you? If so, practice this perception today.

Spruce helps you to experience and evaluate self-reflection from different perceptions.

SEPTEMBER 6
Aromatic visualization with Spruce

Sit quietly. Close your eyes. Take three slow, relaxed, deep breaths. Open your eyes. Put a drop of Spruce on a tissue and inhale the aroma through your nose. Pause and inhale again. Visualize a beautiful garden. As you enjoy walking in this early Autumn garden, notice that you are drawn to a body of still water. It might be a little pond or a tiny puddle. Approach this clear water, lean over, and look at your reflection. As you observe, dip your finger in the water, stirring it a bit, and ask to be shown a reflection of your False Self. As the water becomes still again, what do you see? What aspects of yourself are revealed in this image? How do you feel? Stir the water once more, and ask to see the reflection of your True Self. What appears? How do you feel? Stir it one more time and gaze at your Familiar Self. How do you feel about this image? What thoughts come to you? Take some time reflecting upon what was revealed and notice if anything particular has come to your attention. Notice the differences among the images.

Spruce helps you to self-reflect and identify aspects of different states of consciousness.

SEPTEMBER 7
Aromatic prayer with Spruce

Sit quietly. Close your eyes. Take three slow, relaxed, deep breaths. Open your eyes. Put a drop of Spruce on a tissue and inhale the aroma through your nose. Pause and inhale again. Pray out loud or internally: "Dear God, as I reflect upon who I am in the world, may I see my reflection through Your eyes. May I be a reflection of Your grace. May I be a reflection of Your love. May I reflect You in everything I am and everything I do. Amen."

Spruce helps you to reflect upon and be aware of God's grace within you.

Fir

Best essential oil for self-understanding.

> *Without self-knowledge, without*
> *understanding the working and*
> *functions of his machine, man cannot*
> *be free, he cannot govern himself and*
> *he will always remain a slave.*
> –Georges Gurdjieff

LATIN NAME: *Abies balsamea*

EXTRACTED FROM: Needles

PSYCHOLOGICAL PROPERTIES: Uplifts. Warms and stabilizes
the emotions.

SUBTLE PROPERTIES: Promotes self-understanding. Heightens
awareness and increases intuition. Associated with the
seal in the animal kingdom.

SEPTEMBER 8
Aromatic affirmation with Fir

Sit quietly. Close your eyes. Take three slow, relaxed, deep
breaths. Open your eyes. Put a drop of Fir on a tissue and
inhale the aroma through your nose. Pause and inhale again.
Say out loud or internally the following affirmation: "With
every experience, every day, I understand who I am."

Fir helps to support your ongoing process of self-
understanding.

Aromatic emotional self-discovery with Fir

Sit quietly. Close your eyes. Take three slow, relaxed, deep breaths. Open your eyes. Put a drop of Fir on a tissue and inhale the aroma through your nose. Pause and inhale again. Ask yourself the following questions and jot down your answers and reflections on a piece of paper.

- What does "self-understanding" mean to me?
- What do I understand about myself?
- What helps me to understand myself?
- In what areas do I need more self-understanding?
- How does growing in self-understanding benefit me?

Inhale the aroma of Fir again and intend that you are breathing in the ability to understand yourself well. Review your answers to the above questions. Reflect and jot down any additional notes.

Fir helps you to experience self-understanding and explore its dynamics in your life.

Aromatic attracting ceremony with Fir

Sit quietly. Close your eyes. Take three slow, relaxed, deep breaths. Open your eyes. Put a drop of Fir on a tissue and inhale the aroma through your nose. Pause and inhale again.

Light a candle. Experience the radiant light of this candle filling you with the ability to understand yourself—compassionately and nonjudgmentally. Know that this understanding is deep and complete, and serves your highest good. Once again, inhale Fir from the tissue and allow your body, mind, heart, and spirit to embrace the ability to understand yourself with a loving heart.

Fir helps you to experience and embody compassionate self-understanding.

SEPTEMBER 11
Aromatic blessing with Fir

Sit quietly. Close your eyes. Take three slow, relaxed, deep breaths. Open your eyes. Put a drop of Fir on a tissue and inhale the aroma through your nose. Pause and inhale again. Say out loud or internally the following blessing: "Bless my willingness to recognize that every experience is an opportunity for growth in self-understanding. Bless the process of self-understanding as it matures into compassion, healing, and wisdom."

Fir helps you to develop self-understanding and to appreciate the blessings of the process.

SEPTEMBER 12
Aromatic activity with Fir

Sit quietly. Close your eyes. Take three slow, relaxed, deep breaths. Open your eyes. Put a drop of Fir on a tissue and inhale the aroma through your nose. Pause and inhale again.

Think of a part of your life in which you would like to experience greater self-understanding. Close your eyes, relax, and imagine that you are sitting in a comfortable movie theater. Allow a "movie" to appear on the screen. As you watch, know that you are being shown something that will assist you, in a gentle way, to further your self-understanding. Discover what this "movie" is telling you about yourself. What are you being shown? How does this enhance your self-understanding? Spend some time with this "movie" and learn what you can from it, at this moment. Now inhale Fir again and gently tap your forehead three times with the fingertips of your dominant hand, imagining that you are gently directing this understanding deep into your consciousness. Then rest your fingers on your forehead and know that this information is being integrated on all levels—body, mind, heart, and spirit. Finally, breathe deeply and feel your body relax into a peaceful sense of increased understanding and appreciation of yourself.

Fir helps you to experience greater insights for self-understanding.

SEPTEMBER 13
Aromatic visualization with Fir

Sit quietly. Close your eyes. Take three slow, relaxed, deep breaths. Open your eyes. Put a drop of Fir on a tissue and inhale the aroma through your nose. Pause and inhale again. Visualize a beautiful garden. In the east side of this Autumn garden, discover an exquisite, tall pillar of vines. The vines are flourishing and growing upward. This draws your attention to the sky above you. As you look up into the sky, what do you see? Is it day or night? What is the weather like? Are there clouds? Is it sunny? How are you affected by the state of the sky? Now, make some changes to it. Do you want to alter the weather? If so, what would you do? How would this affect you? Do you want to change the color? How would this affect you? Go ahead and make any changes you desire and notice how each change affects you. Design a sky exactly as you would like it. Now, sit down and rest against the pillar of vines. Look upward at the sky that you have created. Spend some time here to understand how you feel beneath this new sky.

Fir helps you to understand yourself and how you might be affected by changes in the outer world.

SEPTEMBER 14
Aromatic prayer with Fir

Sit quietly. Close your eyes. Take three slow, relaxed, deep breaths. Open your eyes. Put a drop of Fir on a tissue and inhale the aroma through your nose. Pause and inhale again. Pray out loud or internally: "Divine One, as I come to understand myself, may I understand You. You are the center of my being and the source of my life. In knowing who I am, may I come to know myself as Yours. Amen."

Fir helps you to grow in understanding yourself, in your relationship with the Divine.

Bay Laurel

Best essential oil for using good judgment.

Property may be destroyed and money
may lose its purchasing power;
but character, health, knowledge,
and good judgment will always be
in demand under all conditions.
    –Roger Babson

LATIN NAME: *Laurus nobilis*

EXTRACTED FROM: Leaves

PSYCHOLOGICAL PROPERTIES: Warms the emotions. Promotes mental clarity. Relieves stress.

SUBTLE PROPERTIES: Promotes and supports using good judgment. Promotes prophetic visions and intuition. Clears the mind. Associated with the elephant in the animal kingdom.

SEPTEMBER 15
Aromatic affirmation with Bay Laurel

Sit quietly. Close your eyes. Take three slow, relaxed, deep breaths. Open your eyes. Put a drop of Bay Laurel on a tissue and inhale the aroma through your nose. Pause and inhale again. Say out loud or internally the following affirmation: "Every day I use good judgment to the best of my ability."

Bay Laurel helps you to use good judgment in your daily activities.

SEPTEMBER 16
Aromatic emotional self-discovery with Bay Laurel

Sit quietly. Close your eyes. Take three slow, relaxed, deep breaths. Open your eyes. Put a drop of Bay Laurel on a tissue and inhale the aroma through your nose. Pause and inhale again. Ask yourself the following questions and jot down your answers and reflections on a piece of paper.

- ⤙ What does "using good judgment" mean to me?
- ⤙ When have I used good judgment?
- ⤙ When did I fail to use good judgment?
- ⤙ What helps me to use good judgment?
- ⤙ What hinders my using good judgment?
- ⤙ How does using good judgment benefit me?

Inhale the aroma of Bay Laurel again and intend that you are breathing in the ability to use good judgment. Review your answers to the above questions. Reflect and jot down any additional notes.

Bay Laurel helps you to use good judgment, and to understand its dynamics in your life.

SEPTEMBER 17
Aromatic integrating ceremony with Bay Laurel

Sit quietly. Close your eyes. Take three slow, relaxed, deep breaths. Open your eyes. Put a drop of Bay Laurel on a tissue and inhale through your nose. Pause and inhale again. Pour some water into a glass. Hold the glass of water with both hands and intend that it is imbued with light and the ability to use good judgment. As you drink the water, think: "I am filled with light and the capacity to use good and wise judgment." When you have finished drinking, experience this feeling at a deep level, especially as it pertains to your life experiences and personal truth.

Bay Laurel helps you to embody the ability to use good judgment.

SEPTEMBER 18
Aromatic blessing with Bay Laurel

Sit quietly. Close your eyes. Take three slow, relaxed, deep breaths. Open your eyes. Put a drop of Bay Laurel on a tissue and inhale the aroma through your nose. Pause and inhale again. Say out loud or internally the following blessing: "Bless all the ways in which I use good judgment. Bless all that supports my using good judgment. Bless all the experiences in my life that call for good judgment, so I might become ever more skillful in its use."

Bay Laurel helps you to use good judgment and to understand its blessings in your life.

SEPTEMBER 19
Aromatic activity with Bay Laurel

Have a piece of paper and a pen ready. Sit quietly. Close your eyes. Take three slow, relaxed, deep breaths. Open your eyes. Put a drop of Bay Laurel on a tissue and inhale the aroma through your nose. Pause and inhale again. Remember a time when you used good judgment to make a decision. It could have been for something relatively routine, like deciding to eat a healthy snack or deciding to put some time aside to exercise. It could have been for something more significant such as deciding where to live or which job to take. On the piece of paper at the top, write a name for this situation in which you used good judgment. Now, begin listing all the factors that contributed to the process. Consider your thoughts and your feelings, and those of friends and family. Decide if there were physical, relationship, and spiritual factors involved. What about your personal values? Timing? Finances? Now review your list. Can you discover anything about yourself as you look at the process you went through to use good judgment? Inhale Bay Laurel again and notice if you would add to or change your list in any way. Take some time to reflect upon what you have discovered about yourself as a person who uses good judgment.

Bay Laurel helps you to use good judgment and to understand the process you go through for using good judgment.

SEPTEMBER 20
Aromatic visualization with Bay Laurel

Sit quietly. Close your eyes. Take three slow, relaxed, deep breaths. Open your eyes. Put a drop of Bay Laurel on a tissue and inhale the aroma. Pause and inhale again. Visualize a beautiful garden. In one area of this Autumn garden is a stunning, large Bay Laurel tree. A gentle breeze wafts its captivating aroma toward you. From behind the tree, a being emerges and approaches you. It might be a human, an animal, or simply a form. As it comes closer, you are aware that this being is your prophetic self—the part of you that is a visionary who discerns truth, beauty, and goodness in yourself and your environment. Greet this being and notice that it is holding out to you a crown of woven Bay Laurel leaves. With thanks, place this crown upon your head and allow yourself to draw in and embrace the gifts of prophetic vision and awareness with a connected and expanded mind. Notice how the garden is touched and affected by the being's presence. Thank this being, and as you watch it leave the garden, reflect upon or imagine what you are able to "see" with the gift of prophetic vision.

Bay Laurel helps you to experience prophetic vision and to understand its gifts.

SEPTEMBER 21
Aromatic prayer with Bay Laurel

Sit quietly. Close your eyes. Take three slow, relaxed, deep breaths. Open your eyes. Put a drop of Bay Laurel on a tissue and inhale the aroma through your nose. Pause and inhale again. Pray out loud or internally: "Holy Spirit, You who sees all and in all ways, help me to expand my own vision. Help me to 'see' what You want me to 'see.' May all that I 'see' help me to serve You more fully and help me to walk with ever more integrity on my true path. Amen."

Bay Laurel helps you to experience prophetic visions in service to the Divine.

Clary Sage

Best essential oil for intuition.

> *Intuition isn't the enemy,*
> *but the ally, of reason.*
> –John Kord Lagemann

LATIN NAME: *Salvia sclarea*

EXTRACTED FROM: Flowering plant

PSYCHOLOGICAL PROPERTIES: Promotes a sense of well-being. Relaxes and eases nervous tension and panic.

SUBTLE PROPERTIES: Develops and supports intuition. Strengthens the "inner eye," helping us to "see" more clearly. Increases dreaming. Promotes insights. Associated with the archangel Jeremiel in the angelic realm and the snake in the animal kingdom.

SEPTEMBER 22
Aromatic affirmation with Clary Sage

Sit quietly. Close your eyes. Take three slow, relaxed, deep breaths. Open your eyes. Put a drop of Clary Sage on a tissue and inhale the aroma through your nose. Pause and inhale again. Say out loud or internally the following affirmation: "I am intuitive. I value my intuition. I use my intuition."

Clary Sage helps to promote intuition and clear "inner sight."

Aromatic emotional self-discovery with Clary Sage

Sit quietly. Close your eyes. Take three slow, relaxed, deep breaths. Open your eyes. Put a drop of Clary Sage on a tissue and inhale the aroma through your nose. Pause and inhale again. Ask yourself the following questions and jot down your answers and reflections on a piece of paper.

- What does "intuition" mean to me?
- How do I experience intuition in my life?
- How do I access my intuition?
- Do I honor the information that I receive intuitively?
- Am I comfortable or uncomfortable with intuitive information?
- How do I benefit from my intuition?

Inhale the aroma of Clary Sage again and intend that you are breathing in the ability to access your intuition. Review your answers to the above questions. Reflect and jot down any additional notes.

Clary Sage helps you to access your intuition and to understand its dynamics in your life.

Aromatic manifesting ceremony with Clary Sage

Sit quietly. Close your eyes. Take three slow, relaxed, deep breaths. Open your eyes. Find or create an object that represents "dreaming" to you. It might be a dream journal, a picture of clouds, or a drawing of an image that has come to you in a dream. Set it in front of you. Put a drop of Clary Sage on a tissue and inhale through your nose. Pause and inhale again. Hold your hands over or around the object as you send the intention of having intuitive and insightful dreams. This is especially useful when you are in need of receiving guidance through your dreams. From now on, whenever you see, touch, or remember that object, you will be able to connect with your ability to have and understand intuitive dreams. If you choose, place the object in a special place as a reminder.

Clary Sage helps you to manifest intuitive, insightful dreams that can be especially useful for receiving guidance.

SEPTEMBER 25
Aromatic blessing with Clary Sage

Sit quietly. Close your eyes. Take three slow, relaxed, deep breaths. Open your eyes. Put a drop of Clary Sage on a tissue and inhale the aroma through your nose. Pause and inhale again. Say out loud or internally the following blessing: "Bless my intuition, inner visions, and sacred dreams. Bless the information I receive and the guidance I am given. May they serve the highest good for all."

Clary Sage helps you to experience your intuition and inner visions and to discover how they can guide and teach you.

Aromatic activity with Clary Sage

Sit quietly. Close your eyes. Take three slow, relaxed, deep breaths. Open your eyes. Put a drop of Clary Sage on a tissue and inhale the aroma through your nose. Pause and inhale again. Be aware of your whole body. Remember a time when you had an intuitive experience. Let the memory become as vivid as present-moment reality. As you remember, scan your body and become aware of a place in your body that resonates with this experience. Place your hand comfortably on this place and gently breathe, slowly, into the area, letting it expand and contract. Is there a color associated with the experience? Are there words that come to mind? Do images present themselves? Are there any sounds? Discover a bit more about this particular intuitive experience and your physical connection to it.

Clary Sage helps you to experience and understand the dimensions of your intuition.

Aromatic visualization with Clary Sage

Sit quietly. Close your eyes. Take three slow, relaxed, deep breaths. Open your eyes. Put a drop of Clary Sage on a tissue and inhale the aroma through your nose. Pause and inhale again. Visualize a beautiful garden. This is your dream garden. What would you dream about here, now? What have you, in the past, dreamed about in this garden? What have you dreamed about doing? What have you dreamed about having? With whom have you dreamed about spending time? What dreams would you like to come true? Now, explore this place. Pick out one aspect of the garden that represents one of your dreams. What message does it have for you? What insights does it offer? Sit now in this garden and allow yourself to dream for as long as you like.

Clary Sage helps you to dream as well as to understand messages from your dreams.

SEPTEMBER 28
Aromatic prayer with Clary Sage

Sit quietly. Close your eyes. Take three slow, relaxed, deep breaths. Open your eyes. Put a drop of Clary Sage on a tissue and inhale the aroma through your nose. Pause and inhale again. Pray out loud or internally: "Holy Spirit, I give thanks for the intuitive information that You give to me. Help me to receive this information with care and wisdom. May I follow Your counsel, always. Amen."

Clary Sage helps you to receive divine intuitive information and visions that are for your highest good.

End-of-the-Month Days

SEPTEMBER 29

Write an aromatic affirmation for self-reflection and self-understanding

In a small glass container, mix together:

> 3 drops Spruce for self-reflection
> 3 drops Fir for self-understanding
> 6 drops Bay Laurel for good judgment

Have a pen and paper ready. Sit quietly. Close your eyes. Take three slow, relaxed, deep breaths. Open your eyes. Put a drop of your blend on a tissue and inhale the aroma through your nose. Pause and inhale again. Prepare to write an affirmation for self-reflection and self-understanding. Be clear about your intention. Now write a positive statement about you that describes having already achieved that intention in body, mind, heart, and spirit, as if it is already a reality—for example, "I know and understand who I am." Allow your affirmation to come sincerely from within. Be as specific as possible. Read it out loud and put it in a place to see throughout the day. Read it often today.

SEPTEMBER 30
Aromatic ceremony to honor Autumn

Make a blend to honor Autumn. In a small glass container, mix together:

> 1 drop Fir for self-understanding
> 1 drop Roman Chamomile for forgiveness
> 7 drops Lavender for healing on all levels
> 1 drop Jasmine for gratitude
> 2 drops Rose for compassion and unconditional love

Gather five objects that represent the Autumn harvest for you. These could be a variety of squashes, colorful gourds, stalks of corn, or dried leaves. Choose a place in your home where you can create an "Autumn arrangement" to enjoy for the season. Now, sit or stand comfortably in front of the place where you will be arranging your Autumn objects. Place a few drops of your Autumn blend on a tissue and inhale the aroma through your nose. Pause and inhale again. Choose one object. As you place it in the arrangement, say out loud or internally, "I enjoy harvesting all the fruits of self-understanding." Now choose a second, and place it with intention, saying, "I enjoy harvesting all the fruits of forgiveness." With the third, say, "I enjoy harvesting all the fruits of healing." For the fourth, say, "I enjoy harvesting all the fruits of gratitude." And lastly, for the fifth, say, "I enjoy harvesting all the fruits of compassion and unconditional love." Inhale your blend again and allow yourself to embody and radiate the gifts of the Autumn season. Whenever you look at this arrangement, know that your body, mind, heart, and spirit will be experiencing the fruits of the harvest. If at any time you want to rearrange the pieces or add something more, do so knowing that you are continuing to reap the benefits of the season.

❧ October ☙

October is the second Autumn month—a time for moving forward from self-reflection and understanding to self-acceptance, forgiveness, and healing. The essential oils for this month are Palmarosa for self-acceptance, Roman Chamomile for forgiveness, Marjoram for healing grief, Lavender for healing on all levels, and Champaca for receptivity to spiritual guidance.

Palmarosa

Best essential oil for self-acceptance.

> *I define comfort as self-acceptance.*
> *When we finally learn that self-care*
> *begins and ends with ourselves,*
> *we no longer demand sustenance*
> *and happiness from others.*
> –Jennifer Louden

LATIN NAME: *Cymbopogon martini*

EXTRACTED FROM: Flowering plant

PSYCHOLOGICAL PROPERTIES: Uplifts yet calms. Refreshes and clarifies the mind.

SUBTLE PROPERTIES: Promotes self-acceptance. Encourages you to be kind to yourself. Assists any healing process—physical, mental, emotional, or spiritual. Associated with the dragonfly in the animal kingdom.

OCTOBER 1

Aromatic affirmation with Palmarosa

Sit quietly. Close your eyes. Take three slow, relaxed, deep breaths. Open your eyes. Put a drop of Palmarosa on a tissue and inhale the aroma through your nose. Pause and inhale again. Say out loud or internally the following affirmation: "I accept myself as I am—perfectly imperfect. I accept my shortcomings as well as my virtues."

Palmarosa helps you to accept yourself, just as you are.

OCTOBER 2

Aromatic emotional self-discovery with Palmarosa

Sit quietly. Close your eyes. Take three slow, relaxed, deep breaths. Open your eyes. Put a drop of Palmarosa on a tissue and inhale the aroma through your nose. Pause and inhale again. Ask yourself the following questions and jot down your answers and reflections on a piece of paper.

- What does "self-acceptance" mean to me?
- What do I accept about myself? Why?
- What do I struggle to accept about myself? Why?
- What can I do to be more self-accepting?
- How does accepting myself, just as I am, benefit me?

Inhale the aroma of Palmarosa through your nose again and intend that you are breathing in a sense of complete self-acceptance. Review your answers to the above questions. Reflect and jot down any additional notes.

Palmarosa helps you to experience and understand the dynamics of self-acceptance in your life.

Aromatic clearing ceremony with Palmarosa

While standing comfortably with your feet slightly apart, close your eyes. Take three slow, relaxed, deep breaths. Open your eyes. Put a drop of Palmarosa on a tissue and inhale the aroma through your nose. Pause and inhale again. With your dominant hand, make three counterclockwise (up on the left, down on the right) circles in front of your forehead, then your heart, and finally your stomach area, without touching. Then raise your hand in front of your mouth and blow forcefully across your palm with the intention that you are clearing away anything that hinders accepting yourself fully and completely. Inhale Palmarosa again. Feel self-acceptance enliven you.

Palmarosa helps you to experience self-acceptance and to clear away all that hinders it.

OCTOBER 4
Aromatic blessing with Palmarosa

Sit quietly. Close your eyes. Take three slow, relaxed, deep breaths. Open your eyes. Put a drop of Palmarosa on a tissue and inhale the aroma through your nose. Pause and inhale again. Say out loud or internally: "Bless all the virtues and shortcomings that contribute to my unique being. Bless my strengths and my weaknesses. Bless my willingness to accept myself as I am. Bless this journey of self-acceptance that leads me to wholeness."

Palmarosa helps you to accept yourself completely—both the light and the shadow aspects of your being.

OCTOBER 5
Aromatic activity with Palmarosa

Gather together: a piece of writing paper and a pen, colored paints, crayons, or pencils, and a piece of unlined paper large enough for a drawing. Sit comfortably. Put a drop of Palmarosa on a tissue and inhale the aroma through your nose. Pause and inhale again. On the writing paper, make two lists: 1) things you accept about yourself and 2) things you have trouble accepting about yourself. Assign each item on your lists a specific color. You might have different colors for each item, or two or more items might share the same color. Now draw a big circle on your drawing paper and begin to draw inside the circle with each of the colors you have chosen. You might draw patterns, a detailed image, a landscape, or a person. Do not pay attention to whether or not this is "art" but rather, like a child, let your imagination guide your hand as you put the colors into the circle. When complete, look at this drawing and begin to reflect upon what each of the various colors add, as well as how they create something together. What do you feel when you look at this colorful drawing? Intend that, with this activity, you have a greater ability to accept, work with, and create with all of the "colors" of you. Know that this acceptance is being developed and integrated into your being in body, mind, heart, and spirit.

Palmarosa helps you to experience self-acceptance, knowing that all aspects of who you are contribute separately and collectively to your uniqueness.

OCTOBER 6
Aromatic visualization with Palmarosa

Sit quietly. Close your eyes. Take three slow, relaxed, deep breaths. Open your eyes. Put a drop of Palmarosa on a tissue and inhale the aroma through your nose. Pause and inhale again. Visualize a beautiful garden. Observe what this Autumn garden is like this time of year. Notice that there are plants in full bloom and others, such as annuals and early-blooming perennials, that are already beginning to lose their vitality. Perhaps you remove a few dried leaves or a wilted flower. Reflect upon how this living, natural garden is not "perfect." There may be spots that are bare or overgrown. There may be areas that are dry and colorless. Let yourself fully appreciate the uniqueness of this Autumn garden, which is different from the gardens of Spring and Summer. Acknowledge that each season has its own form of beauty and notice how you are able to accept and appreciate this. Discover that the imperfections are part of what makes this natural garden real and authentic. Recognize how this relates to you and helps you to accept yourself completely.

Palmarosa helps you to accept the authentic beauty of the imperfections in the outer world and your inner world.

Aromatic prayer with Palmarosa

Sit quietly. Close your eyes. Take three slow, relaxed, deep breaths. Open your eyes. Put a drop of Palmarosa on a tissue and inhale the aroma through your nose. Pause and inhale again. Pray out loud or internally: "Holy One, may I love and accept myself as You love and accept me. May I be kind to myself as You are kind to me. May I open more fully to Your presence and understanding. Amen."

Palmarosa helps you to experience self-acceptance through acknowledging divine acceptance.

Roman Chamomile

Best essential oil for forgiveness.

> *To err is human, to forgive divine.*
> –Alexander Pope

LATIN NAME: *Anthemis nobilis*

EXTRACTED FROM: Flowering plant

PSYCHOLOGICAL PROPERTIES: Calms. Relaxes. Eases anxiety, anger, and fear.

SUBTLE PROPERTIES: Promotes forgiveness and emotional healing. Promotes inner peace, patience, and understanding. Helps to release past resentments. Associated with the canary in the animal kingdom.

OCTOBER 8
Aromatic affirmation with Roman Chamomile

Sit quietly. Close your eyes. Take three slow, relaxed, deep breaths. Open your eyes. Put a drop of Roman Chamomile on a tissue and inhale the aroma through your nose. Pause and inhale again. Say out loud or internally the following affirmation: "I am able to forgive. I forgive others who have hurt me. I forgive myself for my faults."

Roman Chamomile helps you to experience forgiveness of others and yourself.

OCTOBER 9

Aromatic emotional self-discovery with Roman Chamomile

Sit quietly. Close your eyes. Take three slow, relaxed, deep breaths. Open your eyes. Put a drop of Roman Chamomile on a tissue and inhale the aroma through your nose. Pause and inhale again. Ask yourself the following questions and jot down your answers and reflections on a piece of paper.

- ↤ What does "forgiveness" mean to me?
- ↤ Have I been able to truly forgive in the past? If so, what was it?
- ↤ Is there something I want to forgive myself for? If so, what is it?
- ↤ Is there someone I need to forgive? If so, who and why?
- ↤ What prevents me from being able to forgive?
- ↤ How does being able to forgive benefit me?

Inhale the aroma of Roman Chamomile through your nose again and intend that you are breathing the ability to forgive. Review your answers to the above questions. Reflect and jot down any additional notes.

Roman Chamomile helps you to experience forgiveness and to understand its dynamics in your life.

Aromatic attracting ceremony with Roman Chamomile

Sit quietly. Close your eyes. Take three slow, relaxed, deep breaths. Open your eyes. Put a drop of Roman Chamomile on a tissue and inhale through your nose. Pause and inhale again. Light a candle. Imagine the radiant light of this candle filling you, from head to toe, with a sense of "forgiveness"—for yourself and others. Allow yourself to rest in this feeling for as long as you like. Notice how the light embraces your heart, helping you to forgive what you are ready to forgive. If there is any other place in your body that particularly needs or wants the light, let it focus in that area now. Inhale Roman Chamomile once again. Sense forgiveness in your body, mind, heart, and spirit.

Roman Chamomile helps you to experience forgiveness when you are emotionally ready.

Aromatic blessing with Roman Chamomile

Sit quietly. Close your eyes. Take three slow, relaxed, deep breaths. Open your eyes. Put a drop of Roman Chamomile on a tissue and inhale the aroma through your nose. Pause and inhale again. Say out loud or internally: "Bless the power and blessings of forgiveness—peace, freedom, acceptance, empowerment, integrity, and compassion. Bless the opportunities in my life to experience genuine forgiveness that help me to grow in character."

Roman Chamomile helps you to experience the power and blessings of forgiveness.

OCTOBER 12
Aromatic activity with Roman Chamomile

Sit comfortably. Take three slow, relaxed, deep breaths. Put a drop of Roman Chamomile on a tissue and inhale the aroma through your nose. Pause and inhale again. Imagine that you are facing a large, blank wall—eight feet high and twenty feet wide. Give the wall a color. What color did you choose? On the wall, picture a situation that you resent. Know that you are sitting a "safe" distance from this image. Now imagine dividing the wall into two images—you are on one side and the resentful situation is on the other. Notice there is a rope, which represents your emotional connection, linking the two parts of the wall. Is there a place on your body to which the rope attaches? Continue looking at the wall and inhale Roman Chamomile again. Move your dominant hand in a quick upward motion to sever the rope between the two images. Inhale Roman Chamomile again and make a quick downward motion with your hand so the two ends of the rope release from the images and completely dissolve. Now notice the images on the wall. How have they changed? Allow the wall to become blank again, and assign it a color. Is the color the same as before or different? What does this mean to you? Know that there will be shifts in your thoughts and feelings regarding this situation due to the release process you have just experienced.

Roman Chamomile helps you to release your emotional connection and attachment to situations you resent, allowing them to become part of the past.

OCTOBER 13

Aromatic visualization with Roman Chamomile

Sit quietly. Close your eyes. Take three slow, relaxed, deep breaths. Open your eyes. Put a drop of Roman Chamomile on a tissue and inhale the aroma through your nose. Pause and inhale again. Visualize a beautiful garden. Explore this Autumn garden. Notice that leaves have fallen and plants have lost their vitality. Imagine bringing a large quantity of mulch into the garden and begin carefully spreading it around to protect and support the plants as they prepare for Winter. As you do this, think about the people and experiences in your life that were difficult, but that you were able to forgive and release. Realize how this helped you to move onto the next phase of your life. Be grateful for the times and ways you have forgiven, and the healing that resulted. Imagine that your ability to forgive and let go is a "fertilizing mulch" for experiences to come—a rich and nurturing mixture that tends to your beautiful inner garden.

Roman Chamomile helps you to forgive, and to understand and acknowledge how it helps you prepare for further personal growth.

OCTOBER 14

Aromatic prayer with Roman Chamomile

Sit quietly. Close your eyes. Take three slow, relaxed, deep breaths. Open your eyes. Put a drop of Roman Chamomile on a tissue and inhale the aroma through your nose. Pause and inhale again. Pray out loud or internally: "Loving God, forgive me for all the ways in which I need forgiving. Help me to receive Your divine forgiveness. Help me to forgive myself. Help me to forgive others as You have forgiven me. Amen."

Roman Chamomile helps you to both give and receive forgiveness.

Marjoram

Best essential oil for healing grief.

> *Have courage for the great sorrows*
> *of life and patience for the small ones;*
> *and when you have laboriously*
> *accomplished your daily task,*
> *go to sleep in peace. God is awake.*
> –Victor Hugo

LATIN NAME: *Origanum majorana*

EXTRACTED FROM: Flowering plant

PSYCHOLOGICAL PROPERTIES: Calms. Warms and comforts.
Relieves stress, irritability, and mild depression.

SUBTLE PROPERTIES: Helps to heal the heart of grief.
Promotes acceptance of deep emotional loss.
Associated with the gazelle in the animal kingdom.

OCTOBER 15
Aromatic affirmation with Marjoram

Sit quietly. Close your eyes. Take three slow, relaxed, deep breaths. Open your eyes. Put a drop of Marjoram on a tissue and inhale the aroma through your nose. Pause and inhale again. Say out loud or internally the following affirmation: "I am healed from grief in my body, mind, heart, and spirit. I have gently let it go."

Marjoram helps you to gently release grief from your entire being, when you are ready to do so.

Aromatic emotional self-discovery with Marjoram

Sit quietly. Close your eyes. Take three slow, relaxed, deep breaths. Open your eyes. Put a drop of Marjoram on a tissue and inhale the aroma through your nose. Pause and inhale again. Ask yourself the following questions and jot down your answers and reflections on a piece of paper.

> ⤙ What does "grief" mean to me?
>
> ⤙ How do I experience grief?
>
> ⤙ Am I now grieving in my life? If so, about what?
>
> ⤙ Is it time for me to let go and heal this grief? If so, why? If not, why?
>
> ⤙ What is needed to help me heal this grief?
>
> ⤙ How will I benefit from the healing of my grief?

Inhale the aroma of Marjoram again and intend that you are breathing in a sense that your grief is healing and you are able to let it go. Review your answers to the above questions. Reflect and jot down any additional notes.

Marjoram helps you to experience or imagine the healing of grief in your life, and to understand its dynamics.

Aromatic integrating ceremony with Marjoram

Sit quietly. Close your eyes. Take three slow, relaxed, deep breaths. Open your eyes. Put a drop of Marjoram on a tissue and inhale the aroma through your nose. Pause and inhale again. Pour some water into a glass. Hold the glass of water with both hands and intend that it is imbued with light and the ability for your emotional wounds to heal. As you drink, think: "I am filled with light that heals my emotional wounds." When you have finished drinking, experience a sense of emotional freedom and peace.

Marjoram helps you to experience and integrate the peacefulness that comes from emotional healing, especially of grief and loss.

OCTOBER 18
Aromatic blessing with Marjoram

Sit quietly. Close your eyes. Take three slow, relaxed, deep breaths. Open your eyes. Put a drop of Marjoram on a tissue and inhale the aroma through your nose. Pause and inhale again. Say out loud or internally the following blessing: "Bless my willingness to feel grief and loss. Bless my ability, in the right time and way, to allow my grief and loss to heal. Bless all that supports my healing and helps me find peace in my heart."

Marjoram helps you to experience the willingness and ability to heal emotionally.

OCTOBER 19
Aromatic activity with Marjoram

Sit quietly. Close your eyes. Take three slow, relaxed, deep breaths. Open your eyes. Put a drop of Marjoram on a tissue and inhale the aroma through your nose. Pause and inhale again. Put your hands on top of each other and lay them on your chest, over your heart. Take a slow, deep breath in and imagine your emotional wounds healing. As you exhale, intend that your emotional wounds gently leave your body, mind, heart, and spirit. Breathe in a sense of acceptance. Breathe out loneliness. Breathe in a sense of emotional connection. Breathe out grief. Breathe in a sense of healing. Breathe out loss. Continue to inhale positive life force, healing, and love. Continue to breathe out grief, loss, loneliness, and emotional wounds. Inhale the aroma of Marjoram again. Feel a sense of emotional healing, assisted by Marjoram and conscious breathing. Know that this technique is available to you whenever you need it.

Marjoram helps you to allow the healing and release of emotional wounds.

OCTOBER 20
Aromatic visualization with Marjoram

Sit quietly. Close your eyes. Take three slow, relaxed, deep breaths. Open your eyes. Put a drop of Marjoram on a tissue and inhale the aroma through your nose. Pause and inhale again. Visualize a beautiful garden. Be aware of how this Autumn garden has gone through all the cycles of the seasons—the fading of older plants, the emptiness of Winter, the planting of new seeds, the bursting forth of new life, and the fullness of Summer. This beautiful garden wisely accepts the natural cycles of creation and passing away, joy and grief, harvest and emptiness. Now find a comfortable place where you can lie down on the earth. As you lie there, imagine that the wisdom of nature and the earth itself begins to absorb your grief, emotional pain, and loss. Let the healing earth receive all the emotional wounds you are able to release. Know that this beautiful garden is a powerful place that can tend to your deepest hurts. Take some time to just "be" and receive the healing support of this garden.

Marjoram helps you to accept times of loss and grief as part of life's natural cycles.

OCTOBER 21
Aromatic prayer with Marjoram

Sit quietly. Close your eyes. Take three slow, relaxed, deep breaths. Open your eyes. Put a drop of Marjoram on a tissue and inhale the aroma through your nose. Pause and inhale again. Pray out loud or internally: "Dear God, help me to understand that I am never alone—that You are always with me, even in times of deep emotional loss. Take my grief into Your sacred heart and transform it. Hold my wounds to Your holy breast and heal them. Help me to experience Your presence in every moment and within every emotion. Amen."

Marjoram helps you to experience emotional healing with God's presence and comforting love, even when you are in the most painful of emotional places.

Lavender

Best essential oil for healing on all levels. Embodies the spirit of Autumn.

> *Of one thing I am certain,*
> *the body is not the measure of*
> *healing—peace is the measure.*
> –George Melton

LATIN NAME: *Lavandula vera/officinalis*

EXTRACTED FROM: Flowering plant

PSYCHOLOGICAL PROPERTIES: Uplifts. Relaxes. Helps to balance mood swings. Relieves nervous tension and anxiety.

SUBTLE PROPERTIES: Promotes healing on all levels—physical, mental, emotional, and spiritual. Encourages compassion, acceptance, and reconciliation. Associated with the archangel Raphael in the angelic realm and the bear in the animal kingdom.

OCTOBER 22
Aromatic affirmation with Lavender

Sit quietly. Close your eyes. Take three slow, relaxed, deep breaths. Open your eyes. Put a drop of Lavender on a tissue and inhale the aroma through your nose. Pause and inhale again. Say out loud or internally the following affirmation: "I am healed. I am whole."

Lavender assists you with healing on all levels—body, mind, heart, and spirit—leading to acceptance and wholeness.

OCTOBER 23
Aromatic emotional self-discovery with Lavender

Sit quietly. Close your eyes. Take three slow, relaxed, deep breaths. Open your eyes. Put a drop of Lavender on a tissue and inhale the aroma through your nose. Pause and inhale again. Ask yourself the following questions and jot down your answers and reflections on a piece of paper.

- What does "healing" mean to me?
- When have I experienced healing?
- How does healing feel to me?
- What now needs healing in my life?
- How can this healing be accomplished?
- How do I benefit from healing?

Inhale the aroma of Lavender again and intend that you are breathing in a sense of healing. Review your answers to the above questions. Reflect and jot down any additional notes.

Lavender helps you to experience a sense of healing on all levels, and to understand its dynamics in your life.

Aromatic manifesting ceremony with Lavender

Sit quietly. Close your eyes. Take three slow, relaxed, deep breaths. Open your eyes. Find or create an object that represents the process of "healing" for you. This might be a medical symbol, a picture of someone who appears happy and healthy, or a particularly meaningful book. Set it in front of you. Put a drop of Lavender on a tissue and inhale through your nose. Pause and inhale again. Hold your hands over or around the object as you send the intention of healing into it. From now on, whenever you see, touch, or remember that object, the blessing of knowing you are in the process of healing on all levels—body, mind, heart, and spirit—will be with you. If you choose, place the object in a special place as a reminder.

Lavender helps you to experience the process of healing on all levels, and supports you in becoming whole.

Aromatic blessing with Lavender

Sit quietly. Close your eyes. Take three slow, relaxed, deep breaths. Open your eyes. Put a drop of Lavender on a tissue and inhale the aroma through your nose. Say out loud or internally: "Bless all the healing that I have received, am now receiving, and will receive in my life. Bless all that assists me in my journey toward wholeness."

Lavender helps you to experience the blessings and process of healing.

Aromatic activity with Lavender

Sit comfortably. Take a few relaxing breaths. Put a drop of Lavender on a tissue and inhale the aroma through your nose. Pause and inhale again. Lift your arms to the heavens and imagine a lavender-colored light flowing from the depth of the universe. Use your hands to guide this light into the top of your head. Now, move your hands to guide this light through your body. As it flows, imagine it encasing your spinal column—aligning your spine, balancing your energy, and attuning you to a state of wholeness. Imagine this lavender light healing every aspect of your being. Then guide the light to connect you to the core of the earth. As you open your eyes, experience how you are connected to the healing energies of heaven and earth. Lift your arms to the heavens once again and guide this beautiful light into your heart. Lay your hands, one on top of the other, over your heart. Hold them there for as long as you like. Know that whenever you want to experience a sense of healing, you can guide the lavender light into your being.

Lavender helps you to experience the healing energies of spirit and matter.

OCTOBER 27
Aromatic visualization with Lavender

Sit quietly. Close your eyes. Take three slow, relaxed, deep breaths. Open your eyes. Put a drop of Lavender on a tissue and inhale the aroma through your nose. Pause and inhale again. Visualize a beautiful garden. As you look around, reflect upon the word "heal." It comes from the ancient word *haelan*, which means "to make whole." Take some time in this Autumn garden, engaging all of your senses. Notice what you see, the temperature of the air, and the feel of the ground beneath your feet. Look at the sky and experience the weather. What sounds do you hear? What aromas do you smell? Ask yourself: "What makes this garden whole? What elements define its wholeness? Are there any that could be added or taken away that would improve this garden?" Enjoy this garden, and reflect upon how it relates to you and your unique experience and expression of wholeness.

Lavender helps you to experience a state of healing and wholeness, and to understand that many things contribute to it.

OCTOBER 28
Aromatic prayer with Lavender

Sit quietly. Close your eyes. Take three slow, relaxed, deep breaths. Open your eyes. Put a drop of Lavender on a tissue and inhale the aroma through your nose. Pause and inhale again. Pray out loud or internally: "Great Healer, You who have created all in Your perfect image, may I be healed and made whole. Please help me accept and heal all that needs healing in me, so that I may be complete in You. Amen."

Lavender helps you to experience healing, acceptance, and wholeness from a spiritual perspective.

OCTOBER 29
Write an aromatic affirmation for forgiveness and healing

In a small glass container, mix together:

> 2 drops Palmarosa for self-acceptance
> 4 drops Roman Chamomile for forgiveness
> 6 drops Lavender for healing on all levels

Have a pen and paper ready. Sit quietly. Close your eyes. Take three slow, relaxed, deep breaths. Open your eyes. Put a drop of your blend on a tissue and inhale the aroma through your nose. Pause and inhale again. Prepare to write an affirmation for forgiveness and emotional healing. Be clear about your intention. Now write a positive statement about yourself that describes having already achieved that intention in body, mind, heart, and spirit, as if it is already a reality—for example, "I forgive. I am forgiven. My wounded heart is healed." Allow your affirmation to come sincerely from within. Be as specific as possible. Read it out loud and put it in a place to see throughout the day. Read it often today.

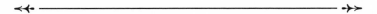

Aromatic activity to prepare a place in your home for quietude

Make a blend for meditation. In a small glass container, mix together:

> 1 drop Roman Chamomile for forgiveness
> 8 drops Lavender for healing on all levels
> 3 drops Rose for compassion and unconditional love

Sit quietly. Close your eyes. Take three slow, relaxed, deep breaths. Open your eyes. Put a drop of your meditation blend on a tissue and inhale the aroma through your nose. Pause and inhale again. Walk around your home and find a place where you can sit comfortably, undisturbed, for at least ten minutes. It should be a place that you like and is aesthetically pleasing to you. If you cannot find a place that fits this description, create one. This is a place for you to sit, quietly and comfortably, and feel a sense of peace and healing in this Autumn season. Now, inhale the aroma once again and close your eyes. Take three slow, relaxed, deep breaths. For a moment, think about the spirit of the season—forgiveness, acceptance, emotional healing, and the emergence of compassion and unconditional love. Then choose a word that represents a peaceful quality for you, such as "peace," "ease," "comfort," or "home." Inhale your meditation blend again.

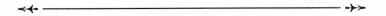

Begin breathing slowly and deeply. Internally say your special word as you inhale and as you exhale. Spend ten minutes gently breathing your special word. At the end of the meditation, inhale your blend once again, knowing that whenever you smell this aroma, you will experience the peaceful quality of your meditation.

OCTOBER 31
New Autumn essential oil: Champaca

Champaca
Best essential oil for receptivity to spiritual guidance.

> *Make known to me your ways, Lord;*
> *teach me your path.*
> *Guide me in your truth and teach me.*
> –Psalm 25:4–5

LATIN NAME: *Michelia champaca*

EXTRACTED FROM: Blossoms

PSYCHOLOGICAL PROPERTIES: Relaxes and produces a euphoric state. Eases stress and inhibition.

SUBTLE PROPERTIES: Promotes intuition and receptivity to spiritual guidance. Balances the energy centers and subtle bodies.

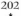

Aromatic visualization exercise with Champaca

Sit quietly. Close your eyes. Take three slow, relaxed, deep breaths. Open your eyes. Put a drop of Champaca on a tissue and inhale the aroma through your nose. Pause and inhale again. Reflect upon an aspect of your life in which you would like spiritual guidance. Perhaps you need to adopt a new perspective, or need support for a difficult situation. Close your eyes again and imagine that you are in a sacred place such as a temple, a church, or a redwood grove. Be sure you are sitting comfortably and fully supported. Using all of your senses as clearly as you can, see where you are, feel the temperature against your skin, notice the quality of light, pay attention to the sounds, and detect any aromas. Notice how your intuition is supported and now opening. Now, ask for spiritual guidance. Wait a few moments. You may see a figure or a vague image, or you may perceive a being of light. Guidance may come as an audible, external voice, an inaudible internal voice, or only as a "feeling." Discover how *your* guidance comes to you now. Welcome this guidance and give thanks. Spend some time being with the information that comes to you. Think of this spiritual guidance as advice from a trustworthy friend who offers their "two cents." It is important that you still make your own decisions and do what is right

for you. Take a few refreshing breaths, and count yourself . . .
1 . . . 2 . . . 3 . . . awake, alert, and present.

Champaca helps to promote intuition and being more
receptive to appropriate spiritual guidance.

ʾ⊰ November ⊱ʾ

November is the last Autumn month—a time to reflect on the many blessings in your life and to be grateful. It is a time for generosity, personal growth, and the development of compassion. The essential oils for this month are Jasmine for gratitude, Cardamom for generosity, Cypress for personal growth, and Rose for compassion and unconditional love.

Jasmine

Best essential oil for gratitude.

> *Gratitude is not only the greatest of virtues, but the parent of all others.*
> –Cicero

LATIN NAME: *Jasminum officinale*

EXTRACTED FROM: Flowers

PSYCHOLOGICAL PROPERTIES: Calms, soothes, and relaxes. Has euphoric properties. Relieves stress and anxiety.

SUBTLE PROPERTIES: Promotes gratitude. Warms and opens the heart center. Helps you to live in and appreciate the present moment. Associated with the archangel Jophiel in the angelic realm and the ladybug in the animal kingdom.

Aromatic affirmation with Jasmine

Sit quietly. Close your eyes. Take three slow, relaxed, deep breaths. Open your eyes. Put a drop of Jasmine on a tissue and inhale the aroma through your nose. Pause and inhale again. Say out loud or internally the following affirmation: "I am grateful for all that is. Gratitude fills my body, mind, heart, and spirit."

Jasmine helps you to experience gratitude on all levels.

Aromatic emotional self-discovery with Jasmine

Sit quietly. Close your eyes. Take three slow, relaxed, deep breaths. Open your eyes. Put a drop of Jasmine on a tissue and inhale the aroma. Pause and inhale again. Ask yourself the following questions and jot down your answers and reflections on a piece of paper.

- What does "being grateful" mean to me?
- What am I grateful for in my life?
- Who am I grateful to have in my life?
- What challenges in the past can I now be grateful for?
- What prevents me from being grateful?
- How does being grateful benefit me?

Inhale the aroma of Jasmine again and intend that you are breathing in a sense of gratitude. Review your answers to the above questions. Reflect and jot down any additional notes.

Jasmine helps you to experience gratitude and to understand its dynamics in your life.

Aromatic clearing ceremony with Jasmine

While standing comfortably with your feet slightly apart, close your eyes. Take three slow, relaxed, deep breaths. Open your eyes. Put a drop of Jasmine on a tissue and inhale the aroma through your nose. Pause and inhale again. With your dominant hand, make three counterclockwise (up on the left, down on the right) circles in front of your forehead, then your heart, and finally your stomach area, without touching. Then raise your hand in front of your mouth and blow forcefully across your palm with the intention that you are releasing anything that prevents you from experiencing a sense of gratitude. Inhale Jasmine again, and embrace a sense of sincere gratitude.

Jasmine helps you to experience gratitude and to clear away any thoughts or feelings that prevent your ability to experience it.

Aromatic blessing with Jasmine

Sit quietly. Close your eyes. Take three slow, relaxed, deep breaths. Open your eyes. Put a drop of Jasmine on a tissue and inhale the aroma through your nose. Pause and inhale again. Say out loud or internally the following blessing: "Bless my life and the gift of life. Bless each precious moment. Bless my ability to experience gratitude as it deepens my capacity to appreciate, celebrate, and honor *all that is.*"

Jasmine helps you to experience the deeper truths, blessings, and teachings of gratitude.

NOVEMBER 5
Aromatic activity with Jasmine

Sit quietly. Close your eyes. Take three slow, relaxed, deep breaths. Open your eyes. Put a drop of Jasmine on a tissue and inhale the aroma through your nose. Pause and inhale again. Take some time to reflect upon the things for which you are grateful. Allow yourself to experience a sensation of "fullness" as gratitude fills your body, mind, heart, and spirit. Write or draw something that represents your gratitude. Sing a song of gratitude. Dance a dance of gratitude. How else could you express or share your gratitude? You might hug someone for whom you are grateful or donate to a charity that once helped you. Find an action that is right for you, and perform it with complete awareness that it is a way of expressing authentic gratitude.

Jasmine helps you to share and express gratitude in creative ways.

Aromatic visualization with Jasmine

Sit quietly. Close your eyes. Take three slow, relaxed, deep breaths. Open your eyes. Put a drop of Jasmine on a tissue and inhale the aroma through your nose. Pause and inhale again. Visualize a beautiful garden. Sit quietly in this end-of-the-season garden, and take some time to reflect upon what it produces for you and the gifts it brings into your life. Think of the visual beauty, the sounds, the aromas, and the peaceful setting that is here for you. As you sit and reflect, feel and speak your gratitude to this garden. Imagine that this garden is receiving, with joy, your appreciation.

Jasmine helps you to be grateful and appreciate all the simple pleasures in your life.

Aromatic prayer with Jasmine

Sit quietly. Close your eyes. Take three slow, relaxed, deep breaths. Open your eyes. Put a drop of Jasmine on a tissue and inhale the aroma through your nose. Pause and inhale again. Pray out loud or internally: "Great Creator, You have given me life. You have guided me every moment. You have held me during the greatest joys and the most difficult challenges. Help me to grow every day in gratitude. Help me to be ever more aware of You and ever more grateful. Amen."

Jasmine helps you to be grateful for your relationship with the Divine.

Cardamom

Best essential oil for generosity.

> ... *true generosity—you give your all,*
> *and yet you always feel*
> *as if it costs you nothing.*
> –Simone de Beauvoir

LATIN NAME: *Elettaria cardamomum*

EXTRACTED FROM: Seeds

PSYCHOLOGICAL PROPERTIES: Uplifts. Warms the emotions. Relieves mild depression. Calms nervousness.

SUBTLE PROPERTIES: Promotes generosity. Expands the capacity for love. Encourages teaching others. Associated with the turkey in the animal kingdom.

NOVEMBER 8
Aromatic affirmation with Cardamom

Sit quietly. Close your eyes. Take three slow, relaxed, deep breaths. Open your eyes. Put a drop of Cardamom on a tissue and inhale the aroma through your nose. Pause and inhale again. Say out loud or internally the following affirmation: "My heart overflows with love for all—ever-expanding, ever-giving, and ever-renewing."

Cardamom helps you to embody and generously express love to those around you.

Aromatic emotional self-discovery with Cardamom

Sit quietly. Close your eyes. Take three slow, relaxed, deep breaths. Open your eyes. Put a drop of Cardamom on a tissue and inhale the aroma through your nose. Pause and inhale again. Ask yourself the following questions and jot down your answers and reflections on a piece of paper.

- What does "being generous" mean to me?
- In what areas of my life have I been generous?
- In what areas of my life has it been harder for me to be generous?
- In what areas of my life have others been generous to me?
- How can I be more generous?
- How does being generous benefit me?

Inhale the aroma of Cardamom again and intend that you are breathing in a sense of generosity. Review your answers to the above questions. Reflect and jot down any additional notes.

Cardamom helps you to experience generosity and to understand its dynamics in your life.

Aromatic attracting ceremony with Cardamom

Sit quietly. Close your eyes. Take three slow, relaxed, deep breaths. Open your eyes. Put a drop of Cardamom on a tissue and inhale the aroma through your nose. Pause and inhale again. Light a candle. Imagine the radiant light of this candle filling your body, mind, heart, and spirit with the capacity for generosity and love. Think about and feel how this affects your relationships, work, and health. Once again, inhale Cardamom from the tissue and embrace the virtuous quality of being generous of spirit.

Cardamom helps you to experience and embody generosity on all levels.

Aromatic blessing with Cardamom

Sit quietly. Close your eyes. Take three slow, relaxed, deep breaths. Open your eyes. Put a drop of Cardamom on a tissue and inhale the aroma through your nose. Pause and inhale again. Say out loud or internally the following blessing: "Bless this universe for its generosity. Bless all my relationships and all my experiences that have been so generous to me. Bless my ability to receive this generosity. Bless my ability to be generous in return."

Cardamom helps you to experience the virtue of generosity and its blessings.

Aromatic activity with Cardamom

Sit quietly. Close your eyes. Take three slow, relaxed, deep breaths. Open your eyes. Put a drop of Cardamom on a tissue and inhale the aroma through your nose. Pause and inhale again. Stand or sit comfortably. Cross your hands and rest them over your heart. Close your eyes and begin to breathe gently, directing your breath into your heart. As you breathe in, imagine that your heart is slowly expanding in its capacity to experience love and to share love with others. With each exhale, move your hands a little bit farther away from your body, sensing the growing vibration of love from your heart. Breathe easily, in and out, until your hands and arms are extended as far as they can reach, in front of you. Become aware of your heart's extraordinary capacity to generate love and to share it. Appreciate the generous nature of your loving heart. Now imagine where you would like to send this love. Make a movement with your arms that sends love out to wherever or whomever you would like it to go.

Cardamom helps you to experience and expand your ability to generously share your love.

Aromatic visualization with Cardamom

Sit quietly. Close your eyes. Take three slow, relaxed, deep breaths. Open your eyes. Put a drop of Cardamom on a tissue and inhale the aroma through your nose. Pause and inhale again. Visualize a beautiful garden. Sit quietly in this Autumn garden, and take some time to reflect upon what it can teach you. What can you learn from the design? The plants? The beauty? The colors? What lessons have you been so generously given as a result of what you see, feel, hear, discover, think, and practice in this special place? Choose one teaching that is particularly helpful or meaningful to you. Imagine that you are generously sharing this teaching with someone in a loving way. Imagine the recipient of this teaching, why you chose them, and how they will benefit.

Cardamom helps you to generously and lovingly give to others by sharing your knowledge.

NOVEMBER 14
Aromatic prayer with Cardamom

Sit quietly. Close your eyes. Take three slow, relaxed, deep breaths. Open your eyes. Put a drop of Cardamom on a tissue and inhale the aroma through your nose. Pray out loud or internally: "You who have created this world and universe with such generous love, teach me to share this love as You do. You who have expressed Your generosity abundantly, may I learn to be as generous in giving of myself in Your name. Amen."

Cardamom helps you to generously serve as an instrument of divine love.

Cypress

Best essential oil for personal growth.

> *It is never too late to become*
> *what you might have been.*
> –George Eliot

LATIN NAME: *Cupressus sempervirens*

EXTRACTED FROM: Twigs

EXTRACTION: Steam distilled

PSYCHOLOGICAL PROPERTIES: Promotes mental clarity.
Emotionally strengthens. Relieves nervous tension.

SUBTLE PROPERTIES: Encourages personal growth.
Strengthens your sense of purpose. Provides support
during change. Associated with the coyote in the
animal kingdom.

NOVEMBER 15
Aromatic affirmation with Cypress

Sit quietly. Close your eyes. Take three slow, relaxed, deep
breaths. Open your eyes. Put a drop of Cypress on a tissue
and inhale the aroma through your nose. Pause and inhale
again. Say out loud or internally the following affirmation:
"I am growing and evolving to be the best I can be."

Cypress helps to encourage personal growth and progress.

NOVEMBER 16
Aromatic emotional self-discovery with Cypress

Sit quietly. Close your eyes. Take three slow, relaxed, deep breaths. Open your eyes. Put a drop of Cypress on a tissue and inhale the aroma through your nose. Pause and inhale again. Ask yourself the following questions and jot down your answers and reflections on a piece of paper.

- ⊷ What does "sense of purpose" mean to me?
- ⊷ What is my purpose at this time in my life?
- ⊷ What areas of my life support my purpose?
- ⊷ What areas of my life do not support my purpose?
- ⊷ How does it benefit me to have a strong sense of purpose?

Inhale the aroma of Cypress again and intend that you are breathing in a strong sense of purpose. Review your answers to the above questions. Reflect and jot down any additional notes.

Cypress helps you to strengthen and understand your sense of purpose.

NOVEMBER 17
Aromatic integrating ceremony with Cypress

Sit quietly. Close your eyes. Take three slow, relaxed, deep breaths. Open your eyes. Put a drop of Cypress on a tissue and inhale the aroma through your nose. Pause and inhale again. Pour some water into a glass. Hold the glass of water with both hands and intend that it is imbued with light and the encouragement to make positive personal changes. As you drink the water, think: "I am growing and changing to be the best person I can be, for the good of all." When you have finished, feel supported in body, mind, heart, and spirit to make the personal changes you would like to make.

Cypress helps you to experience positive personal growth and change.

NOVEMBER 18
Aromatic blessing with Cypress

Sit quietly. Close your eyes. Take three slow, relaxed, deep breaths. Open your eyes. Put a drop of Cypress on a tissue and inhale the aroma through your nose. Pause and inhale again. Say out loud or internally the following blessing: "Bless all the experiences, both challenging and joyful, that help me to grow emotionally and spiritually. Bless all that supports this growth so that I may strongly embrace and fulfill my life's purpose."

Cypress helps you to grow emotionally and spiritually as you strengthen your sense of purpose.

NOVEMBER 19
Aromatic activity with Cypress

Sit quietly. Close your eyes. Take three slow, relaxed, deep breaths. Open your eyes. Put a drop of Cypress on a tissue and inhale the aroma through your nose. Pause and inhale again. Gather the arts and crafts materials needed to create two collages. This can be done with paper images cut from magazines, your own drawings, or items you have around your home. First, create a collection that expresses, "Who I am, now." Next, create a collection that expresses, "Who I am becoming, but not yet." Take some quiet time to observe and reflect upon these two different collections. Notice the feelings, sensations, and thoughts that arise. Inhale Cypress one more time, and then dismantle the two groups to create a third one that contains elements of both. Be aware that you are assisting in growing and integrating your present and future selves with this experience.

Cypress helps you to take the necessary steps to grow into and embody your future self.

NOVEMBER 20
Aromatic visualization with Cypress

Sit quietly. Close your eyes. Take three slow, relaxed, deep breaths. Open your eyes. Put a drop of Cypress on a tissue and inhale the aroma. Pause and inhale again. Visualize a beautiful garden. Be with the simplicity of this end-of-the-season garden. Become aware of the sound of a running stream. It might be in an unexplored part of this garden or it might be in an area that is very familiar. Find this stream of clear, pure water and stand near it as it moves gracefully along. Look downstream and imagine that all that you want to release from your life is moving away from you in the water. Experience a sense of letting go. Now, look upstream and imagine all that enables you to grow, change, and become who you are meant to be is coming toward you. Experience a sense of inviting it all in. Now take a deep breath of the fresh air and notice how you feel.

Cypress helps to support you while you let go what is unneeded, and call in what is needed, to grow emotionally and spiritually.

NOVEMBER 21
Aromatic prayer with Cypress

Sit quietly. Close your eyes. Take three slow, relaxed, deep breaths. Open your eyes. Put a drop of Cypress on a tissue and inhale the aroma through your nose. Pause and inhale again. Pray out loud or internally: "Great Spirit, show me my purpose and how I might best serve You. Help me to remember that You are always with me, supporting me, as I grow stronger in my purpose. Help me to become who You want me to be. Amen."

Cypress helps you to grow into your life purpose with divine support and guidance.

Rose

Best essential oil for compassion and unconditional love.

> *Until he extends his circle*
> *of compassion to include*
> *all living things,*
> *man will not himself find peace.*
> –Albert Schweitzer

LATIN NAME: *Rosa damascena*

EXTRACTED FROM: Blossoms

PSYCHOLOGICAL PROPERTIES: Soothes the emotions. Uplifts the heart. Eases grief and mild depression. Eases negative emotions such as resentment and jealousy.

SUBTLE PROPERTIES: Promotes compassion and unconditional love for others and for self. Heals emotional wounds of the heart. Associated with the archangel Zadkiel in the angelic realm and the dove in the animal kingdom.

NOVEMBER 22
Aromatic affirmation with Rose

Sit quietly. Close your eyes. Take three slow, relaxed, deep breaths. Open your eyes. Put a drop of Rose on a tissue and inhale the aroma through your nose. Say out loud or internally the following affirmation: "My heart is healing. I am a compassionate and loving person."

Rose helps to promote the healing of emotional wounds, allowing you to be a loving person.

NOVEMBER 23
Aromatic emotional self-discovery with Rose

Sit quietly. Close your eyes. Take three slow, relaxed, deep breaths. Open your eyes. Put a drop of Rose on a tissue and inhale the aroma through your nose. Pause and inhale again. Ask yourself the following questions and jot down your answers and reflections on a piece of paper.

- What does "unconditional love" mean to me?
- How do I experience unconditional love?
- In what areas of my life have I experienced unconditional love?
- In what areas of my life do I lack unconditional love?
- Am I able to give as well as receive unconditional love?
- How do I benefit from being able to experience unconditional love?

Inhale the aroma of Rose again and intend that you are breathing in unconditional love. Review your answers to the above questions. Reflect and jot down any additional notes.

Rose helps you to experience unconditional love and to understand its dynamics in your life.

Aromatic manifesting ceremony with Rose

Sit quietly. Close your eyes. Take three slow, relaxed, deep breaths. Open your eyes. Find an object that represents "compassion" for you, such as a picture of a spiritual teacher, a symbol, such as a heart, or a particular book. Set it in front of you. Put a drop of Rose on a tissue and inhale the aroma through your nose. Pause and inhale again. Hold your hands over or around the object as you send the intention of compassion, for yourself and others, into the object. From now on, whenever you see, touch, wear, or remember this object, a sense of compassion will be with you in body, mind, heart, and spirit. If you choose, place the object in a special place as a reminder.

Rose helps you to experience compassion, for yourself and others, on all levels.

Aromatic blessing with Rose

Sit quietly. Close your eyes. Take three slow, relaxed, deep breaths. Open your eyes. Put a drop of Rose on a tissue and inhale the aroma. Pause and inhale again. Say out loud or internally the following blessing: "Bless all that is in need of love. Bless all that is healed by love. Bless all that is transformed by love. Bless the love I receive. Bless the love I give."

Rose helps you to experience and learn the blessing of love in action.

NOVEMBER 26
Aromatic activity with Rose

Sit quietly. Close your eyes. Take three slow, relaxed, deep breaths. Open your eyes. Put a drop of Rose on a tissue and inhale the aroma through your nose. Pause and inhale again. Know that love is literally good for you. The body and mind are positively affected by it. Realize that anyone giving, receiving, or even witnessing an act of love and compassion experiences the benefits of enhanced immune function, and physical and mental relaxation. Today, make a commitment to accomplish three "random acts of kindness" in a loving and compassionate way. This could be for a friend, a spouse, a neighbor, a daughter, or a complete stranger. Remember the "golden rule": "Do unto others as you would have them do unto you." Write your three acts of kindness on a piece of paper and keep it with you as a reminder. As you complete each one, notice what you experience and how you feel in your body, mind, heart, and spirit.

Rose helps you to experience and share love and kindness.

NOVEMBER 27
Aromatic visualization with Rose

Sit quietly. Close your eyes. Take three slow, relaxed, deep breaths. Open your eyes. Put a drop of Rose on a tissue and inhale the aroma through your nose. Pause and inhale again. Visualize a beautiful garden. Begin to walk around this end-of-the-season garden, and find the place that is the "heart." Stand or sit in this heart center and feel it filling your body, mind, heart, and spirit with love. Notice how it nourishes and replenishes the entire garden. Inhale the aroma of Rose again. What do you notice here in the heart of the garden? How do you feel? Spend some time here, and allow your heart and your entire being to receive its blessings.

Rose helps you to experience love at the center of your world and to understand its importance.

NOVEMBER 28
Aromatic prayer with Rose

Sit quietly. Close your eyes. Take three slow, relaxed, deep breaths. Open your eyes. Put a drop of Rose on a tissue and inhale the aroma through your nose. Pray out loud or internally: "Beloved God, You have healed me with your unconditional love and compassion. May I learn to love as You love. Amen."

Rose helps you to experience divine love and healing.

End-of-the-Month Days

NOVEMBER 29
Write an aromatic affirmation for personal growth and gratitude

In a small glass container, mix together:

> 1 drop Cypress for personal growth
> 3 drops Jasmine for gratitude
> 3 drops Cardamom for generosity
> 5 drops Rose for compassion and unconditional love

Have a pen and paper ready. Sit quietly. Close your eyes. Take three slow, relaxed, deep breaths. Open your eyes. Put a drop of your blend on a tissue and inhale the aroma through your nose. Pause and inhale again. Prepare to write an affirmation for personal growth and gratitude. Be clear about your intention. Now write a positive statement about yourself that describes having already achieved that intention in body, mind, heart, and spirit, as if it is already a reality—for example, "I am grateful that I am who I want to be." Allow your affirmation to come sincerely from within. Be as specific as possible. Read it out loud and put it in a place to see throughout the day. Read it often today.

NOVEMBER 30

**Aromatic ceremony to honor your accomplishments this
Autumn**

Choose one of your favorite essential oils among the Autumn
essential oils: Spruce, Fir, Bay Laurel, Clary Sage, Palmarosa,
Roman Chamomile, Marjoram, Lavender, Champaca, Jasmine, Cardamom, Cypress, or Rose. Sit quietly. Close your
eyes. Take three slow, relaxed, deep breaths. Open your eyes.
Put a drop of your chosen oil on a tissue and inhale the
aroma through your nose. Pause and inhale again. Reflect
back upon the past Autumn season and identify your accomplishments. Don't be modest. Notice each and every goal you
have accomplished, from small to large. Inhale your oil once
again, and take a large step forward. As you do, say out loud
or internally, "I have accomplished _____ this Autumn."
Inhale your oil again, and take another step, saying out loud
or internally, "I have also accomplished _____ in these
last few months." With one more step and one final inhalation, say out loud or internally, "I want to be sure I acknowledge accomplishing _____." Now turn around and
visualize looking back at yourself prior to taking these three
steps. Notice how, in only a few minutes, something has
changed within you simply through the process of acknowledging what you have accomplished. Now ask yourself what

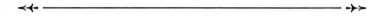

you might like to do to celebrate what you have accomplished. This could be buying a new blank book for journaling, taking a meditation class, or simply planning an afternoon to daydream on the couch with a cup of tea. You may wish to celebrate with a friend. Think of something that would please you and make a commitment to do this for yourself now, to honor your accomplishments this Autumn.

Winter

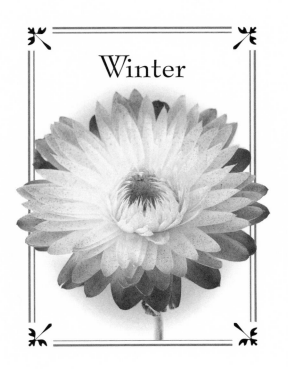

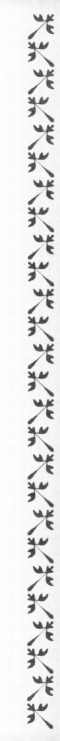

The Winter Months
December, January, February

Winter is the season of the soul that signals rest. It is a time to feel comfortable, safe, and secure—in body, mind, heart, and spirit. A sense of being *home* embraces you. There is an awareness of wholeness, satisfaction, and abundance. It is a time of peace and trust, and in that, there is restoration and rejuvenation. It is a time when increasing wisdom can lead the way to contemplative spirituality. Winter is the season that represents the senior stage of your life.

·❧ December ❧·

December is the first Winter month—a time to feel comfortable, warm, safe, and secure. This well-grounded state helps you to build the inner strength that supports the progression to higher states of consciousness. The essential oils for this month are Benzoin for comfort, Vetiver for feeling safe, Vanilla for a deep connection to Mother Earth, and Oakmoss for a sense of abundance.

Benzoin

Best essential oil for comfort.

> *As long as you derive inner help*
> *and comfort from anything, keep it.*
> –Mahatma Gandhi

LATIN NAME: *Styrax benzoin*

EXTRACTED FROM: Resin

PSYCHOLOGICAL PROPERTIES: Calms. Relieves stress and tension. Eases emotional exhaustion.

SUBTLE PROPERTIES: Comforts, warms, and steadies. Associated with the dog in the animal kingdom.

DECEMBER 1
Aromatic affirmation with Benzoin

Sit quietly. Close your eyes. Take three slow, relaxed, deep breaths. Open your eyes. Put a drop of Benzoin on a tissue and inhale the aroma through your nose. Pause and inhale again. Say out loud or internally the following affirmation: "I am comfortable and at home in my body, my mind, my self, and my life."

Benzoin helps you to experience feeling comfortable and well-grounded.

DECEMBER 2
Aromatic emotional self-discovery with Benzoin

Sit quietly. Close your eyes. Take three slow, relaxed, deep breaths. Open your eyes. Put a drop of Benzoin on a tissue and inhale the aroma through your nose. Pause and inhale again. Ask yourself the following questions and jot your answers and reflections on a piece of paper.

- ↞ What does "being comfortable" mean to me?
- ↞ How do I experience being comfortable in my life?
- ↞ What makes me feel comfortable?
- ↞ What makes me feel uncomfortable?
- ↞ What changes can I make to be more comfortable?
- ↞ How do I benefit from feeling comfortable?

Inhale the aroma of Benzoin again and intend that you are breathing in a deep sense of comfort. Review your answers to the above questions. Reflect and jot down any additional notes.

Benzoin helps you to experience being comfortable and to understand its dynamics in your life.

DECEMBER 3
Aromatic clearing ceremony with Benzoin

While standing comfortably with your feet slightly apart, close your eyes. Take three slow, relaxed, deep breaths. Open your eyes. Put a drop of Benzoin on a tissue and inhale the aroma through your nose. Pause and inhale again. With your dominant hand, make three counterclockwise (up on the left, down on the right) circles in front of your forehead, then your heart, and finally your stomach area, without touching.

Raise your hand to your mouth and blow forcefully across your palm with the intention that you are releasing anything that prevents you from receiving the warmth and stability of authentic comfort.

Benzoin helps you to experience comfort and clear away any thoughts, feelings, beliefs, behaviors, or habits that may hinder it.

DECEMBER 4
Aromatic blessing with Benzoin

Sit quietly. Close your eyes. Take three slow, relaxed, deep breaths. Open your eyes. Put a drop of Benzoin on a tissue and inhale the aroma through your nose. Pause and inhale again. Say out loud or internally the following blessing: "Bless the warmth of community. Bless the steadiness of friendship. Bless the reassurance of family and the comfort of home, as they bless me."

Benzoin helps you to experience comfort in your relationships as they bless your life.

DECEMBER 5
Aromatic activity with Benzoin

Sit quietly. Close your eyes. Take three slow, relaxed, deep breaths. Open your eyes. Put a drop of Benzoin on a tissue and inhale the aroma through your nose. Pause and inhale again. Find a place in your home that is especially comfortable for you. Notice what it is about this place that gives you these wonderful feelings of comfort and warmth. Is it the colors? The furniture? The view from a window? The memories? Is there anything that you could add or remove that would make it even more comfortable? Take some time to make this place a bit more cozy and comfortable, if you choose. Enjoy consciously spending some time here and notice how you feel.

Benzoin helps you to experience comfort at home and to understand what it is in your environment that is comforting for you.

DECEMBER 6
Aromatic visualization with Benzoin

Sit quietly. Close your eyes. Take three slow, relaxed, deep breaths. Open your eyes. Put a drop of Benzoin on a tissue and inhale the aroma through your nose. Pause and inhale again. Visualize a beautiful garden. As you begin wandering through this Winter garden, notice what you are wearing. Discover how you have chosen the perfect clothing to keep you warm, comfortable, and protected in this Winter landscape. Do you have on warm socks, boots, and gloves? A big coat with a hood? A scarf? A woolen hat? Notice how your inner wisdom knows how to provide what comforts and tends to you. Spend some time here and enjoy the garden while staying cozy and warm.

Benzoin helps you to feel comfortable and to understand what it is that you need in order to be comfortable.

Aromatic prayer with Benzoin

Sit quietly. Close your eyes. Take three slow, relaxed, deep breaths. Open your eyes. Put a drop of Benzoin on a tissue and inhale the aroma through your nose. Pause and inhale again. Pray out loud or internally: "Holy Spirit, Divine Comforter, hold me warmly within Your sacred heart and steady in Your love. I am comforted in Your presence. Amen."

Benzoin helps you to experience and connect with the comfort of the Divine.

Vetiver

Best essential oil for feeling safe.

> *This is the true nature of home—*
> *it is the place of peace; the shelter,*
> *not only from injury, but from*
> *all terror, doubt and division.*
> –John Ruskin

LATIN NAME: *Vetiveria zizanioides*

EXTRACTED FROM: Roots

PSYCHOLOGICAL PROPERTIES: Calms. Relaxes. Relieves stress
and tension.

SUBTLE PROPERTIES: Promotes a deep sense of safety and
security. Protects. Encourages a sense of belonging.
Associated with the porcupine in the animal kingdom.

DECEMBER 8
Aromatic affirmation with Vetiver

Sit quietly. Close your eyes. Take three slow, relaxed, deep
breaths. Open your eyes. Put a drop of Vetiver on a tissue
and inhale the aroma through your nose. Pause and inhale
again. Say out loud or internally the following affirmation:
"I am secure, protected, and safe. I am present."

Vetiver helps you to feel safe, secure, and protected.

Aromatic emotional self-discovery with Vetiver

Sit quietly. Close your eyes. Take three slow, relaxed, deep breaths. Open your eyes. Put a drop of Vetiver on a tissue and inhale the aroma through your nose. Pause and inhale again. Ask yourself the following questions and jot down your answers and reflections on a piece of paper.

> ⤙ What does "feeling safe" mean to me?
>
> ⤙ When do I feel safe?
>
> ⤙ When do I not feel safe?
>
> ⤙ What helps me to feel safe?
>
> ⤙ What prevents me from feeling safe?
>
> ⤙ How do I benefit from feeling safe?

Inhale the aroma of Vetiver again and intend that you are breathing in a sense of safety. Review your answers to the above questions. Reflect and jot down any additional notes.

Vetiver helps you to experience feeling safe and to understand its dynamics in your life.

Aromatic attracting ceremony with Vetiver

Sit quietly. Close your eyes. Take three slow, relaxed, deep breaths. Open your eyes. Put a drop of Vetiver on a tissue and inhale the aroma through your nose. Pause and inhale again. Light a candle. Imagine the radiant light of the candle filling your body, mind, heart, and spirit with a strong sense of belonging. Inhale the aroma once again and feel connected and accepted throughout your being.

Vetiver helps you to experience a profound sense of belonging.

DECEMBER 11
Aromatic blessing with Vetiver

Sit quietly. Close your eyes. Take three slow, relaxed, deep breaths. Open your eyes. Put a drop of Vetiver on a tissue and inhale the aroma through your nose. Pause and inhale again. Say out loud or internally: "Bless all that keeps me feeling safe, secure, and protected. Bless all that feeling safe, secure, and protected allows me to be and to do."

Vetiver helps you to feel safe, secure, and protected and to experience the blessings they bring into your life.

DECEMBER 12
Aromatic activity with Vetiver

Sit or stand comfortably. Put a drop of Vetiver on a tissue and inhale the aroma through your nose. Pause and inhale again. Hold your arms out straight on either side of you. Imagine that you are encased and held safely within a caring bubble of protection that extends from head to toe and to the tips of your fingers on both sides. Imagine that it surrounds you—right, left, front, behind, above, and below. Know that this protective bubble allows in, all that protects and sustains you, such as love, blessings, and good will. It keeps out, all that may harm you, such as anger, envy, and prejudice. Be aware that anytime you need or want this sense of protection, you can inhale the aroma of Vetiver, extend your arms, and intend that the protective bubble is around you.

Vetiver helps to protect you from negative influences that may harm you, whether from people, places, things, or situations.

DECEMBER 13
Aromatic visualization with Vetiver

Sit quietly. Close your eyes. Take three slow, relaxed, deep breaths. Open your eyes. Put a drop of Vetiver on a tissue and inhale the aroma through your nose. Visualize a beautiful garden. Imagine walking into this Winter landscape. In the south area, find a beautiful stone. It has exquisite colorations and is perfectly shaped and sized. Touch or hold this stone. Experience its density and solidity. Honor, acknowledge, or appreciate it in some way as a representation of the earth. Let yourself sense how this sacred garden is created, supported, and protected by the earth. Feel these qualities below, above, around, and within this garden. Reflect upon how the earth also provides these qualities for you. Feel a sense of gratitude.

Vetiver helps you to experience feeling safe, supported, and protected here on earth.

Aromatic prayer with Vetiver

Sit quietly. Close your eyes. Take three slow, relaxed, deep breaths. Open your eyes. Put a drop of Vetiver on a tissue and inhale the aroma through your nose. Pause and inhale again. Pray out loud or internally: "Dear God, Your strength and power hold me safe. May I rest in the protection of Your loving arms. May I feel secure in the love of Your holy heart. Amen."

Vetiver helps you to rest in the safety, security, and protection of divine love.

Vanilla

Best essential oil for a deep connection to Mother Earth.

We must learn not to disassociate
the airy flower from the earthy root,
for the flower that is cut off from
its root fades, and its seeds are barren,
whereas the root, secure in mother
earth, can produce flower after flower
and bring their fruit to maturity.
–Kabbalah

LATIN NAME: *Vanilla planifolia*

EXTRACTED FROM: Pods

PSYCHOLOGICAL PROPERTIES: Comforts. Calms and warms the emotions.

SUBTLE PROPERTIES: Promotes a deep connection with Mother Earth. Comforts and warms. Associated with the turtle in the animal kingdom.

DECEMBER 15
Aromatic affirmation with Vanilla

Sit quietly. Close your eyes. Take three slow, relaxed, deep breaths. Open your eyes. Put a drop of Vanilla on a tissue and inhale the aroma through your nose. Pause and inhale again. Say out loud or internally the following affirmation: "I am securely connected with Mother Earth. I am at home and comfortable here on this beautiful and bountiful planet."

Vanilla helps you to experience a deep connection with being at home on earth.

Aromatic emotional self-discovery with Vanilla

Sit quietly. Close your eyes. Take three slow, relaxed, deep breaths. Open your eyes. Put a drop of Vanilla on a tissue and inhale the aroma through your nose. Pause and inhale again. Ask yourself the following questions and jot down your answers and reflections on a piece of paper.

- What does being "deeply connected to Mother Earth" mean to me?
- How do I experience this connection—in body, mind, emotions, and spirit?
- What in my life helps me experience this sense of connectedness?
- What in my life prevents me from experiencing this sense of connectedness?
- How do I benefit from feeling this connectedness to Mother Earth?

Inhale the aroma of Vanilla again and intend that you are breathing in a sense of being comfortable, secure, and connected. Review your answers to the above questions. Reflect and jot down any additional notes.

Vanilla helps you to experience a sense of being connected to the earth on all levels, and to understand its dynamics in your life.

Aromatic integrating ceremony with Vanilla

Sit quietly. Close your eyes. Take three slow, relaxed, deep breaths. Open your eyes. Put a drop of Vanilla on a tissue and inhale the aroma through your nose. Pause and inhale again. Pour some water into a glass. Hold the glass of water with both hands and intend that it is imbued with light and the ability to have a deep connection with Mother Earth. As you drink the water, think: "I am filled with light and a deep connection to the beauty, power, and sustenance of the earth." When you have finished drinking, experience the sense of being strongly connected to and nurtured by earth, your home.

Vanilla helps you to experience and integrate the sense of being present and connected to Mother Earth.

Aromatic blessing with Vanilla

Sit quietly. Close your eyes. Take three slow, relaxed, deep breaths. Open your eyes. Put a drop of Vanilla on a tissue and inhale the aroma through your nose. Pause and inhale again. Say out loud or internally: "Bless this Earth, my Mother, and all the gifts she so generously gives to me. Bless the comfort and sustenance that I draw from her. Bless all that allows me to be connected—fully present, centered, and grounded."

Vanilla helps you to experience the blessings of being truly connected to Mother Earth.

Aromatic activity with Vanilla

Sit comfortably. Close your eyes. Take three slow, relaxed, deep breaths. Open your eyes. Put a drop of Vanilla on a tissue and inhale the aroma through your nose. Pause and inhale again. Hold a piece of bread in your hands. Begin to reflect upon all that is represented in this food. Reflect upon the earth and the elements that enabled the grain to grow—the sun, the rain, and the air. Consider the farmer who grew and harvested this grain. Think about the grain being ground into flour. Reflect upon the people who brought the flour to the bakery where it was made into bread. Think of everyone who contributed to bringing this bread to you and how you are connected to them because of it. Fill your body with gratitude for the bounty of the earth and for all the people who have contributed to your receiving this bounty. Eat this bread, and as you do, imagine that your awareness and gratitude nourish you and make you feel secure and comfortable—in body, mind, heart, and spirit. Consciously receive this nourishment of good food that connects you to the earth and its many gifts.

Vanilla helps you to connect with and receive the comforting, replenishing bounty of the earth and her people.

Aromatic visualization with Vanilla

Sit quietly. Close your eyes. Take three slow, relaxed, deep breaths. Open your eyes. Put a drop of Vanilla on a tissue and inhale the aroma through your nose. Pause and inhale again. Visualize a beautiful garden. Look into the sky, reflecting upon the Winter solstice that is approaching. Notice how it feels to be here in this garden on one of the shortest days and longest nights of the year. Reach down and touch the ground, letting your hands sense the earth resting so peacefully. Send a blessing to the earth. Give thanks to the coming sun. Appreciate your own journey through the luminous darkness and toward the birthing light.

Vanilla helps you to experience a deep connection to the earth and its cycles.

DECEMBER 21
Aromatic prayer with Vanilla

Sit quietly. Close your eyes. Take three slow, relaxed, deep breaths. Open your eyes. Put a drop of Vanilla on a tissue and inhale the aroma through your nose. Pause and inhale again. Pray out loud or internally: "Great Mother Earth, my body is made from you and will return to you. I give thanks for the food you give me for nourishment, for the beauty that nourishes my soul, and for the ability to expand my heart to receive the blessings that comfort my spirit. I love and honor you, dear Earth. Amen."

Vanilla helps you to experience and honor your sacred connection to Mother Earth.

Oakmoss

Best essential oil for a sense of abundance.

> *Life in abundance comes only through great love.*
> –Elbert Hubbard

LATIN NAME: *Evernia prunastri*

EXTRACTED FROM: Moss

PSYCHOLOGICAL PROPERTIES: Calms. Helps to balance the emotions.

SUBTLE PROPERTIES: Promotes a sense of abundance—having what you need to thrive in body, mind, heart, and spirit. Promotes a sense of safety and security. Associated with the buffalo in the animal kingdom.

DECEMBER 22
Aromatic affirmation with Oakmoss

Sit quietly. Close your eyes. Take three slow, relaxed, deep breaths. Open your eyes. Put a drop of Oakmoss on a tissue and inhale the aroma through your nose. Pause and inhale again. Say out loud or internally the following affirmation: "I attract abundance. I receive abundance. I am abundant in all ways."

Oakmoss helps you to feel abundant in body, mind, heart, and spirit.

Aromatic emotional self-discovery with Oakmoss

Sit quietly. Close your eyes. Take three slow, relaxed, deep breaths. Open your eyes. Put a drop of Oakmoss on a tissue and inhale the aroma through your nose. Pause and inhale again. Ask yourself the following questions and jot down your answers and reflections on a piece of paper.

> ⊶ What does "abundance" mean to me?
> ⊶ In what areas of my life do I experience abundance?
> ⊶ What helps me to experience a sense of abundance?
> ⊶ In what areas of my life do I feel a lack of abundance?
> ⊶ What interferes with my experiencing a sense of abundance?
> ⊶ How do I benefit from feeling abundant?

Inhale the aroma of Oakmoss again and intend that you are breathing in a deep sense of abundance. Review your answers to the above questions. Reflect and jot down any additional notes.

Oakmoss helps you to experience abundance and to understand its dynamics in your life.

DECEMBER 24
Aromatic manifesting ceremony with Oakmoss

Sit quietly. Close your eyes. Take three slow, relaxed, deep breaths. Open your eyes. Put a drop of Oakmoss on a tissue and inhale the aroma through your nose. Pause and inhale again. Open your eyes. Find or create an object that represents "abundance" for you. This might be a plate of delicious food, a wallet full of money, or a picture of a group of friends. Set it in front of you. Hold your hands around the object as you send into it the intention of manifesting abundance naturally and easily in your life. From now on, whenever you see, touch, or remember this object, the sense of abundance will be with you in body, mind, heart, and spirit. If you choose, place the object in a special place as a reminder.

Oakmoss helps you to experience feeling fully abundant in your life.

DECEMBER 25
Aromatic blessing with Oakmoss

Sit quietly. Close your eyes. Take three slow, relaxed, deep breaths. Open your eyes. Put a drop of Oakmoss on a tissue and inhale the aroma through your nose. Pause and inhale again. Say out loud or internally: "Bless the abundance of the universe. Bless the gifts that Spirit so generously bestows upon the earth. Bless the abundance that fills my body, mind, heart, and spirit, and bless my ability to receive it."

Oakmoss helps you to experience abundance and its blessings on all levels.

DECEMBER 26
Aromatic activity with Oakmoss

Sit quietly. Close your eyes. Take three slow, relaxed, deep breaths. Open your eyes. Put a drop of Oakmoss on a tissue and inhale the aroma through your nose. Pause and inhale again. Draw or make a collage of a bouquet of flowers. Let your creativity determine the number and type of flowers. When you have finished, imagine that each bloom represents someone or something that contributes to your sense of abundance. Write their name or the description next to the flower. When you are finished, determine if there is anything else you would like to add to your bouquet of abundance, such as something you would like in your life right now. Add the flower and identify it. Place the picture where you can see it. Know that when you see or remember this bouquet, you are affirming the reality of abundance and all that is abundant in your life now and always.

Oakmoss helps you to experience, understand, and expand the abundance in your life.

DECEMBER 27
Aromatic visualization with Oakmoss

Sit quietly. Close your eyes. Take three slow, relaxed, deep breaths. Open your eyes. Put a drop of Oakmoss on a tissue and inhale the aroma through your nose. Pause and inhale again. Visualize a beautiful garden. This garden is abundant with the quiet beauty of Winter. As you walk around this garden, notice a flash of gold on the ground. As you approach it, you find a beautiful gold coin—a symbol of abundance—here in the bareness of Winter. Pick up the coin and discover if there is a picture or writing on the coin. What does it want to communicate to you about abundance? Turn the coin over in your hands, look at it carefully from all sides, and let yourself experience its message. What would you like to do with this coin? Do whatever feels right for you. You may choose to put it back on the ground, put it in your pocket, or keep it in your hand. Before you leave, thank the garden for this gift of abundance to you. Notice what receiving this gold coin means to you in your daily life.

Oakmoss helps you to experience the abundant gifts that are always available to you.

DECEMBER 28
Aromatic prayer with Oakmoss

Sit quietly. Close your eyes. Take three slow, relaxed, deep breaths. Open your eyes. Put a drop of Oakmoss on a tissue and inhale the aroma through your nose. Pause and inhale again. Pray out loud or internally: "God of Light, help me, on this long and dark Winter night, to remember You and Your abundant love. May I feel abundant in You. May I prosper in my devotion to You. Amen."

Oakmoss helps you to experience spiritual abundance that springs from divine love.

End-of-the-Month Days

DECEMBER 29
Write an aromatic affirmation for feeling safe and secure

In a small glass container, mix together:

> 2 drops Vetiver for feeling safe
> 10 drops Vanilla for a deep connection to
> Mother Earth

Have a pen and paper ready. Sit quietly. Close your eyes. Take three slow, relaxed, deep breaths. Open your eyes. Put a drop of your blend on a tissue and inhale the aroma through your nose. Pause and inhale again. Prepare to write an affirmation for feeling safe and secure. Be clear about your intention. Now write a positive statement about yourself that describes having already achieved that intention in body, mind, heart, and spirit, as if it is already a reality—for example, "I am safe and secure. I am home." Allow your affirmation to come sincerely from within. Be as specific as possible. Read it out loud and put it in a place to see throughout the day. Read it often today.

DECEMBER 30
Aromatic activity for protecting your home

Sit quietly. Close your eyes. Take three slow, relaxed, deep breaths. Open your eyes. Put a drop of Vetiver on a tissue

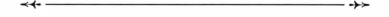

and inhale the aroma through your nose. Pause and inhale again. With the bottle of Vetiver, walk around the perimeter of your house, put a drop of Vetiver at every corner of your house, and say, "My house is protected." Then walk around again and put a drop of Vetiver every three feet, between the corners, as you say, "I am safe at home." Go into your home and inhale the aroma from the tissue again. Now, walk into each room and say with intention and visualization, "This home is safe and secure for all."

DECEMBER 31
Aromatic ceremony to honor Winter

Make a blend to honor Winter. In a small glass container, mix together:

> 1 drop Vetiver for feeling safe
> 2 drops Vanilla for a deep connection to Mother Earth
> 1 drop Myrrh to understand the spiritual perspective of emotional challenges
> 2 drops Rosewood for spiritual opening and growth
> 1 drop Elemi for balancing spiritual and worldly life
> 4 drops Sandalwood for a sense of oneness

Gather in front of you: several strips of paper, a pen, and a small cardboard box. Inhale your Winter blend, and reflect

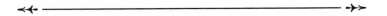

upon Winter as a time of deep rest and preparation for springtime growth. Identify whatever it is that gives you a sense of wholeness, safety, security, peace, home, and one-ness. Write what you have identified on individual strips of paper. When you are ready, inhale your Winter blend again. Fold each piece of paper and put them in the small card-board box. Take the box outside and dig a hole in the earth. Place the box in the hole and cover it with soil. Now fill a glass with water, hold it in your hands, and say, "I am at peace. I am at home. I am at rest. May my hopes and dreams burst forth in this coming Spring." Spend a moment to enjoy the feeling of this affirmation. Now pour the glass of water on the soil that covers your buried cardboard box. Inhale your Winter blend again and say, "I am grateful for all that gives me a sense of peace and wholeness." Know that as the soil rests this Winter, you also rest. Know that all that has been accomplished in the previous seasons is integrating in your body, mind, heart, and spirit, preparing for the creative potential that emerges in Spring.

⁓⤙ January ⤚⁓

January is the second Winter month—a time to rest and be at peace, allowing your spirit to rejuvenate and restore. It is a time to trust, surrender, and be still. The essential oils for this month are: Neroli for a sense of peace, Spikenard for a sense of trust, Myrrh to understand the spiritual perspective of emotional challenges, Rosewood for spiritual opening and growth, and Immortelle for spiritual strength.

Neroli

Best essential oil for a sense of peace.

First keep the peace within yourself,
then you can also
bring peace to others.
–Thomas à Kempis

LATIN NAME: *Citrus aurantium*

EXTRACTED FROM: Blossoms

PSYCHOLOGICAL PROPERTIES: Has slight euphoric properties. Soothes shock. Relieves anxiety, stress, and mild depression.

SUBTLE PROPERTIES: Promotes a sense of peace and wholeness. Rejuvenates and nurtures the heart center. Associated with the goldfish in the animal kingdom.

Aromatic affirmation with Neroli

Sit quietly. Close your eyes. Take three slow, relaxed, deep breaths. Open your eyes. Put a drop of Neroli on a tissue and inhale the aroma through your nose. Pause and inhale again. Say out loud or internally the following affirmation, slowly, three times: "I am at peace. I am a person of peace."

Neroli helps you to experience and embody a sense of peace.

Aromatic emotional self-discovery with Neroli

Sit quietly. Close your eyes. Take three slow, relaxed, deep breaths. Open your eyes. Put a drop of Neroli on a tissue and inhale the aroma through your nose. Pause and inhale again. Ask yourself the following questions and jot down your answers and reflections on a piece of paper.

-+ What does "being at peace" mean to me?
-+ What makes me feel at peace?
-+ What disturbs my sense of peace?
-+ How does peacefulness affect my body? Mind? Heart? Spirit?
-+ How does being at peace benefit me?

Inhale the aroma of Neroli again and intend that you are breathing in a sense of peace. Review your answers to the above questions. Reflect and jot down any additional notes.

Neroli helps you to experience a sense of peace and to understand its dynamics in your life.

Aromatic clearing ceremony with Neroli

While standing comfortably with your feet slightly apart, close your eyes. Take three slow, relaxed, deep breaths. Open your eyes. Put a drop of Neroli on a tissue and inhale the aroma through your nose. Pause and inhale again. With your dominant hand, make three counterclockwise (up on the left, down on the right) circles in front of your forehead, then your heart, and finally your stomach area, without touching. Then raise your hand in front of your mouth and blow forcefully across your palm with the intention that you are releasing anything that interferes with your experiencing and embracing a sense of peace.

Neroli helps you to experience a sense of peace and to release what hinders it.

Aromatic blessing with Neroli

Sit quietly. Close your eyes. Take three slow, relaxed, deep breaths. Open your eyes. Put a drop of Neroli on a tissue and inhale the aroma through your nose. Pause and inhale again. Say out loud or internally the following blessing: "Bless the peace that nurtures my soul, heals my mind, replenishes my heart, and uplifts my spirit. Bless all that peace teaches and gives to me. May the peace that I experience be a blessing to all."

Neroli helps you to experience the blessings and wisdom of peace, and to share it with others.

Aromatic activity with Neroli

While standing comfortably with your feet slightly apart, close your eyes. Take three slow, relaxed, deep breaths. Open your eyes. Put a drop of Neroli on a tissue and inhale the aroma through your nose. Pause and inhale again. Now place your hands in prayer position in front of your heart (palms together, fingers pointing upward). As you inhale, move your arms out to the side, straightening and moving upward in a big circle that brings your hands and palms together again in prayer position over your head. When you exhale, allow your hands to drop down, stopping once again in front of your heart. Repeat this nine times. With every inhalation, have the intention that you are gathering the peacefulness of Spirit into your arms, and as you exhale, have the intention that you bring this peace into your body and let it rest within your heart.

Neroli helps you to gather a sense of peace that nurtures and fills your heart.

Aromatic visualization with Neroli

Sit quietly. Close your eyes. Take three slow, relaxed, deep breaths. Open your eyes. Put a drop of Neroli on a tissue and inhale the aroma through your nose. Pause and inhale again. Visualize a beautiful garden. As you experience this Winter garden, notice what aspects of it bring you a sense of peace. Allow yourself to wander through the landscape and experience it with all of your senses—seeing, hearing, feeling, smelling, and even tasting the Winter air on your tongue. Is there anything that you would like to change about this garden to make it more peaceful? Is there something to remove, add, or alter in some way? Make any changes you desire to enhance the peacefulness of this garden. Feel yourself embrace this peace, and rest here for as long as you like.

Neroli helps you to experience and create a sense of peace.

JANUARY 7
Aromatic prayer with Neroli

Sit quietly. Close your eyes. Take three slow, relaxed, deep breaths. Open your eyes. Put a drop of Neroli on a tissue and inhale the aroma through your nose. Pause and inhale again. Pray out loud or internally: "Dear God, may I be filled with Your peace, the peace that *passeth understanding.* May I become a being of peace and contribute to Your peace on Earth. Amen."

Neroli helps you to experience a sense of peace and to act peacefully in accordance with the Divine.

Spikenard

Best essential oil for a sense of trust.

For it is mutual trust,
even more than mutual interest that
holds human associations together.
–H. L. Mencken

LATIN NAME: *Nardostachys jatamansi*

EXTRACTED FROM: Root

PSYCHOLOGICAL PROPERTIES: Useful as a meditation oil.
Relieves stress and tension. Calms restlessness.

SUBTLE PROPERTIES: Restores a sense of trust and faith.
Comforts and brings peace to the heart center,
especially when facing the predicaments of the world.
Associated with the cricket in the animal kingdom.

JANUARY 8
Aromatic affirmation with Spikenard

Sit quietly. Close your eyes. Take three slow, relaxed, deep
breaths. Open your eyes. Put a drop of Spikenard on a tissue and inhale the aroma through your nose. Pause and
inhale again. Say out loud or internally the following affirmation: "I trust myself. I know who and what I can trust. I
have faith in my ability to know what is trustworthy."

Spikenard helps you to experience and support a sense of
trust.

Aromatic emotional self-discovery with Spikenard

Sit quietly. Close your eyes. Take three slow, relaxed, deep breaths. Open your eyes. Put a drop of Spikenard on a tissue and inhale the aroma through your nose. Pause and inhale again. Ask yourself the following questions and jot down your answers and reflections on a piece of paper.

- What does "trust" mean to me?
- What makes someone or something trustworthy?
- What makes someone or something not worthy of trust?
- What do I trust? What do I mistrust?
- How does being able to trust appropriately benefit me?

Inhale the aroma of Spikenard again and intend that you are breathing in a renewed sense of trust. Review your answers to the above questions. Reflect and jot down any additional notes.

Spikenard helps you to experience appropriate trust and to understand its dynamics in your life.

Aromatic attracting ceremony with Spikenard

Sit quietly. Close your eyes. Take three slow, relaxed, deep breaths. Open your eyes. Put a drop of Spikenard on a tissue and inhale the aroma through your nose. Pause and inhale again. Light a candle. Imagine the radiant light of this candle filling you completely with a strong sense of trust and faith—in your body, mind, heart, and spirit. Allow it to permeate your entire being.

Spikenard helps you to experience a sense of trust and faith, and the feeling of well-being that it brings.

Aromatic blessing with Spikenard

Sit quietly. Close your eyes. Take three slow, relaxed, deep breaths. Open your eyes. Put a drop of Spikenard on a tissue and inhale the aroma through your nose. Pause and inhale again. Say out loud or internally: "Bless all that helps me to trust. Bless all that challenges me to trust. Bless the gift of trust and faith that heals and brings peace to my heart."

Spikenard helps you to experience a sense of trust and faith, and the blessings they bring into your life.

Aromatic activity with Spikenard

Gather together the ingredients you will need to prepare an enjoyable meal for yourself. Sit quietly. Close your eyes. Take three slow, relaxed, deep breaths. Open your eyes. Put a drop of Spikenard on a tissue and inhale the aroma through your nose. Pause and inhale again. Begin to prepare your meal. As you go through the various stages of preparation, notice and reflect upon each one. Think about how the ingredients are being chopped, sliced, or pulled apart and then combined and mixed together. Smell the aromas as they are being cooked and as their flavors commingle. When you eat this dish, be aware of all the steps that have brought you to enjoy this nourishing and delicious food. What is your experience? Did you trust that the process of chopping and mixing would yield something delicious? Did you have faith that you would enjoy the blend of the tastes and textures?

Spikenard helps you to trust your ability and willingness to take the various steps needed to bring about a positive outcome.

JANUARY 13
Aromatic visualization with Spikenard

Sit quietly. Close your eyes. Take three slow, relaxed, deep breaths. Open your eyes. Put a drop of Spikenard on a tissue and inhale the aroma through your nose. Pause and inhale again. Visualize a beautiful garden. Find or create a devotional place here to honor Spirit. Would you like to place a statue or a picture somewhere? Would you like to build a fountain or a labyrinth? Perhaps you would like a particular arrangement of plants or flowers? Do whatever feels right for you and realize that you are making a place where you can release any of the sorrows or frustrations you might have about the state of the world, your community, your family, or yourself. Let this be a place of devotion in which you replenish your trusting and empathic heart. When you complete your place of devotion, feel yourself filled with a strong sense of trust and renewed faith. Release the burdens of the world, and turn them over to Spirit.

Spikenard helps you to experience a sense of trust that allows you to gently release the burdens you feel about the predicament of the world.

JANUARY 14
Aromatic prayer with Spikenard

Sit quietly. Close your eyes. Take three slow, relaxed, deep breaths. Open your eyes. Put a drop of Spikenard on a tissue and inhale the aroma through your nose. Pause and inhale again. Pray out loud or internally: "Dear God, may my heart be filled with a sense of complete trust and peace. Help me to remember that Your holy hand is ever present, even in the most challenging times. Help me turn my troubles over to You. Teach me to place my trust and faith in You. Amen."

Spikenard helps you to grow in trust and devotion to the Divine.

Myrrh

Best essential oil to understand the spiritual perspective of emotional challenges.

> *Cherish your own emotions*
> *and never undervalue them.*
> –Robert Henri

LATIN NAME: *Commiphora myrrha*

EXTRACTED FROM: Resin

PSYCHOLOGICAL PROPERTIES: Cools heated emotions such as anger and jealousy. Counteracts apathy.

SUBTLE PROPERTIES: Helps to understand the spiritual perspective of emotional challenges. Strengthens a spiritual journey. Promotes emotional harmony and peace. Associated with the archangel Sandalphon in the angelic realm and the deer in the animal kingdom.

JANUARY 15
Aromatic affirmation with Myrrh

Sit quietly. Close your eyes. Take three slow, relaxed, deep breaths. Open your eyes. Put a drop of Myrrh on a tissue and inhale the aroma through your nose. Pause and inhale again. Say out loud or internally the following affirmation: "I experience the Divine in every aspect of my life. In understanding my emotional challenges from a spiritual perspective, I grow in wisdom."

Myrrh helps you to understand your emotional challenges from a spiritual perspective.

Aromatic emotional self-discovery with Myrrh

Sit quietly. Close your eyes. Take three slow, relaxed, deep breaths. Open your eyes. Put a drop of Myrrh on a tissue and inhale the aroma through your nose. Pause and inhale again. Ask yourself the following questions and jot down your answers and reflections on a piece of paper.

> ⊷ What does "emotional challenge" mean to me?
>
> ⊷ How do I experience emotional challenges?
>
> ⊷ How do emotional challenges relate to spirituality?
>
> ⊷ How do I find peace in the midst of challenging times?
>
> ⊷ How does understanding an emotional challenge from a spiritual perspective benefit me?

Inhale the aroma of Myrrh again and intend that you understand your emotional challenges from a spiritual perspective. Review your answers to the above questions. Reflect and jot down any additional notes.

Myrrh helps you to experience and understand emotional challenges as a natural part of life and a natural part of spiritual growth and development.

Aromatic integrating ceremony with Myrrh

Sit quietly. Close your eyes. Take three slow, relaxed, deep breaths. Open your eyes. Put a drop of Myrrh on a tissue and inhale the aroma through your nose. Pause and inhale again. Pour some water into a glass. Hold the glass of water with both hands and intend that it is imbued with light and spiritual wisdom for facing emotional challenges. As you drink the water, think: "I am being gently and slowly filled with light and the spiritual wisdom needed to understand my emotional challenges." When you have finished drinking the water, feel your body, mind, heart, and spirit embrace this sense of spiritual wisdom.

Myrrh helps you to understand emotional challenges from a spiritual perspective.

Aromatic blessing with Myrrh

Sit quietly. Close your eyes. Take three slow, relaxed, deep breaths. Open your eyes. Put a drop of Myrrh on a tissue and inhale the aroma through your nose. Pause and inhale again. Say out loud or internally: "Bless every moment in my life that has helped me with my spiritual journey. Bless every challenge that I have faced. Bless the perfection of every step."

Myrrh helps you to move forward and bless every step you take on your spiritual journey.

Aromatic activity with Myrrh

Sit quietly. Close your eyes. Take three slow, relaxed, deep breaths. Open your eyes. Put a drop of Myrrh on a tissue and inhale the aroma through your nose. Pause and inhale again. On a large piece of paper, draw a line across it that represents your life—from the moment of your birth to the present. Mark the line in five-year sections, leaving plenty of room in each section to write and/or draw. Reflect back upon your life thus far, and put a star on your life line to represent every time you experienced a noteworthy emotional challenge. Above each star, briefly describe the challenge. Complete this part of the activity and then sit back and review the line and its account of emotional trials. Inhale Myrrh once again. Allow yourself to discover and visualize the spiritual lesson of each incident on the life line. Below the star, write in that spiritual lesson, and then draw an image that represents it. When you are finished, look at your life line and see how your spirit can utilize your emotional challenges to help you grow and move forward in your spiritual journey.

Myrrh helps you to perceive and understand the spiritual lessons of difficult times.

Aromatic visualization with Myrrh

Sit quietly. Close your eyes. Take three slow, relaxed, deep breaths. Open your eyes. Put a drop of Myrrh on a tissue and inhale the aroma through your nose. Pause and inhale again.

Visualize a beautiful garden. You have never been to this garden before—it is new to you. Observe and experience this Winter garden for the first time. What stands out to you? Engage your senses of sight, hearing, smell, and touch. Now, allow yourself to connect with the Divine, and then perceive this garden from a spiritual perspective. What do you notice? What particularly stands out? Again, use all of your senses. What can you discover about the difference between a worldly perspective and a spiritual perspective? Notice what you can discover about your spirituality in the simplicity, stillness, and barrenness of this Winter landscape.

Myrrh helps you to observe, experience, and understand the world from a spiritual perspective.

JANUARY 21
Aromatic prayer with Myrrh

Sit quietly. Close your eyes. Take three slow, relaxed, deep breaths. Open your eyes. Put a drop of Myrrh on a tissue and inhale the aroma through your nose. Pause and inhale again. Pray out loud or internally: "Dear God, may I remember that for all my experiences, be they easy or difficult, You are ever with me, and I am ever with You. Amen."

Myrrh helps you to deepen and strengthen your spirituality, as you perceive your life experiences as part of your spiritual journey.

Rosewood

Best essential oil for spiritual opening and growth.

*We are not human beings on a
spiritual journey. We are spiritual
beings on a human journey.*
–Stephen Covey

LATIN NAME: *Aniba rosaeodora*

EXTRACTED FROM: Wood

PSYCHOLOGICAL PROPERTIES: Balances the emotions. Uplifts
the mind. Comforts and warms.

SUBTLE PROPERTIES: Gently balances body, mind, heart, and
spirit for spiritual opening and growth. Calms and
comforts. Associated with the whale in the animal
kingdom.

JANUARY 22
Aromatic affirmation with Rosewood

Sit quietly. Close your eyes. Take three slow, relaxed, deep
breaths. Open your eyes. Put a drop of Rosewood on a tissue and inhale the aroma through your nose. Pause and
inhale again. Say out loud or internally the following affirmation: "Every day, I open and grow in spirit."

Rosewood helps you to gently open to and embrace spiritual growth.

Aromatic emotional self-discovery with Rosewood

Sit quietly. Close your eyes. Take three slow, relaxed, deep breaths. Open your eyes. Put a drop of Rosewood on a tissue and inhale the aroma through your nose. Pause and inhale again. Ask yourself the following questions and jot down your answers and reflections on a piece of paper.

- ⤙ What does "spiritual growth" mean to me?
- ⤙ In what ways have I experienced spiritual growth?
- ⤙ What experiences have led to this growth?
- ⤙ What areas of my life have changed in some way as a result of my spiritual growth?
- ⤙ What can I do to further my spiritual growth?
- ⤙ How do I benefit from spiritual growth?

Inhale the aroma of Rosewood again and intend that you are breathing in a sense of gentle, spiritual opening and growth. Review your answers to the above questions. Reflect and jot down any additional notes.

Rosewood helps you to experience spiritual opening and growth, and to understand its dynamics in your life.

JANUARY 24
Aromatic manifesting ceremony with Rosewood

Sit quietly. Close your eyes. Take three slow, relaxed, deep breaths. Open your eyes. Find or create an object that represents "spiritual growth" to you, such as a spiritual symbol, a statue of a spiritual teacher, or a beautiful picture of nature. Set it in front of you. Put a drop of Rosewood on a tissue and inhale the aroma through your nose. Pause and inhale again. Hold your hands around that object and send the intention of spiritual growth into that object. Hold it close to you. From now on, whenever you see, touch, or remember that object, a sense of unfolding spirituality and growth will be with you in body, mind, heart, and spirit. If you choose, place the object in a special place as a reminder.

Rosewood helps you to move forward and grow on your spiritual journey.

JANUARY 25
Aromatic blessing with Rosewood

Sit quietly. Close your eyes. Take three slow, relaxed, deep breaths. Open your eyes. Put a drop of Rosewood on a tissue and inhale the aroma through your nose. Pause and inhale again. Say out loud or internally: "Bless my ability to be open and receive spiritual sustenance. Bless my growing spirituality and all that has helped me along the way. Bless my body, mind, and heart as I grow in spirit."

Rosewood helps you to grow in spirituality and to understand its blessings in your life.

JANUARY 26
Aromatic activity with Rosewood

Sit quietly. Close your eyes. Take three slow, relaxed, deep breaths. Open your eyes. Put a drop of Rosewood on a tissue and inhale the aroma through your nose. Pause and inhale again. Cut out seven paper circles, making them large enough for you to be able to color. Gather seven crayons or markers—one each of red, orange, yellow, green, blue, purple, and white. Set the circles in front of you, in a vertical row. Color the bottom circle red and imagine that this red is assisting you in strengthening your body as you embrace a sense of security. Going up, color the next circle orange and intend that this color enhances your emotional well-being and creativity. Color the third circle yellow and, as you color, sense it supporting your personal power and integrity. Color the fourth circle green and intend that it is assisting your heart to grow in compassion and love. Color the fifth circle blue and imagine that it helps you to speak your truth. Color the next circle purple and intend that you are activating your intuition. Color the last circle white and intend that it represents your spirituality and connection to the Divine. Now look at these seven colored circles and know that as you created these circles, you were aligning and balancing your energy centers that resonate with these colors. Be aware that as you perform a simple, even playful, action on the "outside" you are also tending to the "inside"—the realm of your imagination, energy, and spirit.

Rosewood helps you to creatively and intentionally balance your energy centers and align them with Spirit. (For more information about your energy centers, see Appendix VI.)

JANUARY 27
Aromatic visualization with Rosewood

Sit quietly. Close your eyes. Take three slow, relaxed, deep breaths. Open your eyes. Put a drop of Rosewood on a tissue and inhale the aroma through your nose. Pause and inhale again. Visualize a beautiful garden. As you begin to stroll through it, become aware how this Winter garden is resting and dormant now. Reflect upon how important it is for this garden to rest, allowing for the rejuvenation that leads to the bursting forth of Spring and Summer. Now, sit quietly in this garden and experience this sense of deep rest. How do you feel? Are you comfortable or uncomfortable in this resting state? Is it familiar or unfamiliar to you? As you rest, ask yourself, "How am I preparing for my spiritual growth?" Allow the answers to come to you. It may be in words, images, or feelings. Reflect on your inner process of preparing for spiritual growth. Take as much time as you want and when you are finished, explore and interact with this special place.

Rosewood helps you to prepare for spiritual growth and to understand the process.

Aromatic prayer with Rosewood

Sit quietly. Close your eyes. Take three slow, relaxed, deep breaths. Open your eyes. Put a drop of Rosewood on a tissue and inhale the aroma through your nose. Pause and inhale again. Pray out loud or internally: "As an acorn grows naturally into an oak tree, may I, Great Spirit, grow more fully and completely into my True Self. May I mature into who You want me to be. Amen."

Rosewood helps you to grow and mature in spirit.

End‑of‑the‑Month Days

JANUARY 29

Write an aromatic affirmation for peace and spiritual understanding

In a small glass container, mix together:

> 2 drops Neroli for a sense of peace
> 1 drop Spikenard for a sense of trust
> 9 drops Myrrh to understand the spiritual
> perspective of emotional challenges

Have a pen and paper ready. Sit quietly. Close your eyes. Take three slow, relaxed, deep breaths. Open your eyes. Put a drop of your blend on a tissue and inhale the aroma through your nose. Pause and inhale again. Prepare to write an affirmation for peace and spiritual understanding. Be clear about your intention. Now write a positive statement about yourself that describes having already achieved that intention in body, mind, heart, and spirit, as if it is already a reality—for example, "I understand life from a spiritual perspective and I am at peace." Allow your affirmation to come sincerely from within. Be as specific as possible. Read it out loud and put it in a place to see throughout the day. Read it often today.

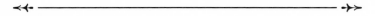

New Winter essential oil: Immortelle

Immortelle (Helichrysum)

Best essential oil for spiritual strength.

> *Humanity is not a gift of nature; it is a*
> *spiritual achievement to be earned.*
> –Richard Bach

LATIN NAME: *Helichrysum italicum*

EXTRACTED FROM: Blossoms

PSYCHOLOGICAL PROPERTIES: Uplifts. Eases mild depression
and nervous exhaustion.

SUBTLE PROPERTIES: Promotes spiritual strength. Integrates
spirituality and compassion. Promotes healing for
emotional wounds.

Aromatic visualization exercise with Immortelle

Sit quietly. Close your eyes. Take three slow, relaxed, deep
breaths. Open your eyes. Put a drop of Immortelle on a tissue and inhale the aroma through your nose. Pause and
inhale again. Bring your awareness to the base of your spine
and imagine a clear red light filling the area, clearing away
anything that weakens and hinders your connection to
Mother Earth. Inhale the aroma again and move your awareness to the area just below your navel and allow a warm

orange light to fill the area, clearing away anything that weakens and hinders your creativity. Inhale the aroma again and move your awareness up to your stomach and imagine a golden yellow light filling the area, clearing away anything that weakens and hinders your personal power and self-confidence. Inhale the aroma again and move your awareness to your heart and allow a beautiful green light to fill the area, clearing away anything that weakens or hinders you from being able to give and receive love. Inhale the aroma again and move your awareness to your throat and imagine a soft blue light filling the area, clearing away anything that weakens or hinders you from knowing and speaking your truth. Inhale the aroma again, and move your awareness to the center of your forehead. Let a deep blue/purple color fill the area, and clear away anything that weakens or hinders your insight and intuition. Inhale the aroma again and, finally, move your attention to the top of your head. Experience a white light radiating there, clearing away anything that weakens or hinders your spiritual wisdom and consciousness. For the last time, inhale the aroma of Immortelle, and intend that anything that weakens your energy and evolution as a spiritual being has been removed. Feel balanced and spiritually strong.

Immortelle helps to promote spiritual strength on all levels as it clears away anything that may hinder it.

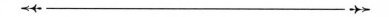

Write an aromatic affirmation for balancing spiritual and worldly life

In a small glass container, mix together:

> 5 drops Rosewood for spiritual opening and growth
>
> 2 drops Cedarwood for a direct connection with the Divine
>
> 3 drops Elemi for balancing spiritual and worldly life
>
> 2 drops Frankincense for spiritual wisdom and consciousness

Have a pen and paper ready. Sit quietly. Close your eyes. Take three slow, relaxed, deep breaths. Open your eyes. Put a drop of your blend on a tissue and inhale the aroma through your nose. Pause and inhale again. Prepare to write an affirmation that will create balance for your spiritual and worldly life. Be clear about your intention. Now write a positive statement about yourself that describes having already achieved that intention in body, mind, heart, and spirit. Write as if your intention is already a reality—for example, "My life is balanced in the spiritual and worldly realms." Allow your affirmation to come sincerely from within. Be as specific as possible. Read it out loud and put it in a place where you will see it throughout the day. Read it often today.

~ February ~

February is the last Winter month—a time to rest in wisdom and wholeness. You shall live balanced in the realm of the physical world and the spiritual world. Your Higher Self—the part of you that is wise and spiritually evolved—experiences a sense of oneness with the Divine. The essential oils for this month are Cedarwood for a direct connection with the Divine, Sandalwood for a sense of oneness, Elemi for balancing spiritual and worldly life, and Frankincense for spiritual wisdom.

Cedarwood

Best essential oil for a direct connection with the Divine.

What we're all striving for
is authenticity,
a spirit-to-spirit connection.
–Oprah Winfrey

LATIN NAME: *Cedrus atlantica*

EXTRACTED FROM: Wood

PSYCHOLOGICAL PROPERTIES: Calms and soothes the mind. Emotionally strengthens. Eases stress and tension.

SUBTLE PROPERTIES: Supports the conscious experience of a direct, strong, certain connection with the Divine. Promotes wisdom. Encourages a calm, meditative state. Associated with the eagle in the animal kingdom.

FEBRUARY 1
Aromatic affirmation with Cedarwood

Sit quietly. Close your eyes. Take three slow, relaxed, deep breaths. Open your eyes. Put a drop of Cedarwood on a tissue and inhale the aroma through your nose. Pause and inhale again. Say out loud or internally the following affirmation: "I am directly connected with the Divine with strength and certainty."

Cedarwood helps you to consciously experience a direct connection with the Divine.

FEBRUARY 2
Aromatic emotional self-discovery with Cedarwood

Sit quietly. Close your eyes. Take three slow, relaxed, deep breaths. Open your eyes. Put a drop of Cedarwood on a tissue and inhale the aroma through your nose. Pause and inhale again. Ask yourself the following questions and jot your answers and reflections down on a piece of paper.

- ← What does "direct connection with the Divine" mean to me?
- ← Have I consciously experienced a direct connection with the Divine?
- ← What would help me to consciously experience a direct connection with the Divine?

➤ What blessings and challenges come with consciously experiencing a direct connection with the Divine?

➤ How do I benefit from knowing and understanding a direct connection with the Divine?

Inhale the aroma of Cedarwood again and intend that you are experiencing a direct connection with the Divine. Review your answers to the above questions. Reflect and jot down any additional notes.

Cedarwood helps you to experience a direct connection with the Divine and to understand its dynamics in your life.

FEBRUARY 3
Aromatic clearing ceremony with Cedarwood

While standing comfortably with your feet slightly apart, close your eyes. Take three slow, relaxed, deep breaths. Open your eyes. Put a drop of Cedarwood on a tissue and inhale the aroma through your nose. Pause and inhale again. With your dominant hand, make three counterclockwise (up on the left, down on the right) circles in front of your forehead, then your heart, and lastly, your stomach area, without touching. Then raise your hand to your mouth and blow forcefully across your palm with the intention that you are releasing whatever hinders your ability to consciously experience a connection with the Divine.

Cedarwood helps you to experience a conscious, direct connection with the Divine and to let go of anything that may hinder it.

Aromatic blessing with Cedarwood

Sit quietly. Close your eyes. Take three slow, relaxed, deep breaths. Open your eyes. Put a drop of Cedarwood on a tissue and inhale the aroma through your nose. Pause and inhale again. Say out loud or internally the following blessing: "Bless my connection with the Divine. Bless the many ways in which I experience my connection with the Divine. Bless this sacred connection as it sustains, guides, and teaches me."

Cedarwood helps you to experience and bless your direct connection with the Divine.

Aromatic activity with Cedarwood

Sit quietly. Close your eyes. Take three slow, relaxed, deep breaths. Open your eyes. Put a drop of Cedarwood on a tissue and inhale the aroma through your nose. Pause and inhale again. Sit comfortably, your hands in prayer position in front of your heart—palms together and fingers pointing upward. Sit with your spine straight and your feet planted comfortably on the floor in front of you. Pay attention to your breath. Notice the movement of your body as you breathe in and breathe out. Breathe awareness into your entire body—head, neck, torso, arms, legs, and feet. Spend the next five minutes gently watching the rise and fall of breath in your body. Intend that with each inhalation, you breathe in serenity and wisdom, and with each exhalation, you relax and let go of stress and tension. If you have a favorite spiritual prayer, poem, song, or affirmation that you would like to say internally or out loud, do so now, and let yourself be filled with its message.

Cedarwood helps you to experience and embrace a calm, relaxed, wise state of mind.

FEBRUARY 6
Aromatic visualization with Cedarwood

Sit quietly. Close your eyes. Take three slow, relaxed, deep breaths. Open your eyes. Put a drop of Cedarwood on a tissue and inhale the aroma through your nose. Pause and inhale again. Visualize a beautiful garden. What is calming and meditative about this Winter garden for you? What would you change or add here to enhance these qualities? Clear an area? Plant a specific type of flower? Create a meditation area? Build a labyrinth? Add a fountain? Make any changes or additions that feel right to you and then spend some time meditating in this garden and connecting with its sacredness.

Cedarwood helps you to experience a meditative state and to understand the qualities that support it for you.

Aromatic prayer with Cedarwood

Sit quietly. Close your eyes. Take three slow, relaxed, deep breaths. Open your eyes. Put a drop of Cedarwood on a tissue and inhale the aroma through your nose. Pause and inhale again. Pray out loud or internally: "Divine Source, open my heart and mind to Your wisdom, Your peace, and Your love. Open my heart and mind, so that I experience a direct connection with You. May this connection grow ever stronger. Amen."

Cedarwood helps you to experience a connection to the Divine in a direct and prayerful way.

Sandalwood

Best essential oil for a sense of oneness.

*Man's ultimate destiny is
to become one with the Divine Power
which governs and sustains
the creation and its creatures.*
–Alfred A. Montapert

LATIN NAME: *Santalum album*

EXTRACTED FROM: Wood

PSYCHOLOGICAL PROPERTIES: Profoundly relaxes. Promotes a
sense of well-being. Soothes nervous tension and
anxiety. Relieves stress.

SUBTLE PROPERTIES: Promotes a sense of oneness and states
of higher consciousness. Promotes mystical
experiences. Associated with the archangel Azrael in
the angelic realm and the cat in the animal kingdom.

FEBRUARY 8
Aromatic affirmation with Sandalwood

Sit quietly. Close your eyes. Take three slow, relaxed, deep
breaths. Open your eyes. Put a drop of Sandalwood on a tissue and inhale the aroma through your nose. Pause and
inhale again. Say out loud or internally the following affirmation: "I am one with the vast universe. I am one with *all
that is.*"

Sandalwood helps you to experience a sense of oneness
and connection with *all that is.*

Aromatic emotional self-discovery with Sandalwood

Sit quietly. Close your eyes. Take three slow, relaxed, deep breaths. Open your eyes. Put a drop of Sandalwood on a tissue and inhale the aroma through your nose. Pause and inhale again. Ask yourself the following questions and jot down your answers and reflections on a piece of paper.

- What does "higher consciousness" mean to me?
- When have I experienced a state of higher consciousness?
- What helps me to experience states of higher consciousness?
- What hinders me from experiencing states of higher consciousness?
- What are the benefits of experiencing states of higher consciousness for me?

Inhale the aroma of Sandalwood again and intend that you are breathing in a state of higher consciousness. Review your answers to the above questions. Reflect and jot down any additional notes.

Sandalwood helps you to experience the realm of higher consciousness and to understand its dynamics in your life.

Aromatic attracting ceremony with Sandalwood

Sit quietly. Close your eyes. Take three slow, relaxed, deep breaths. Open your eyes. Put a drop of Sandalwood on a tissue and inhale the aroma through your nose. Pause and inhale again. Light a candle. Imagine the radiant light of this candle filling you with a strong, peaceful awareness of the oneness of all life. Experience that oneness in your body, mind, heart, and spirit. Allow it to permeate your entire being. Once again, inhale Sandalwood from the tissue. Feel at peace. Feel at one.

Sandalwood helps you to be peacefully and completely at one with yourself and the universe.

Aromatic blessing with Sandalwood

Sit quietly. Close your eyes. Take three slow, relaxed, deep breaths. Open your eyes. Put a drop of Sandalwood on a tissue and inhale the aroma through your nose. Pause and inhale again. Say out loud or internally: "Bless the oneness of all of life. Bless the many playful ways through which oneness is expressed. Bless my life as a complex and unique expression of perfect oneness."

Sandalwood helps you to experience and bless the oneness that underlies all of life.

FEBRUARY 12
Aromatic activity with Sandalwood

Sit quietly. Close your eyes. Take three slow, relaxed, deep breaths. Open your eyes. Put a drop of Sandalwood on a tissue and inhale the aroma. Pause and inhale again. Play a recorded piece of music that promotes a state of higher consciousness for you. Sit or lie down comfortably, and as you inhale Sandalwood again, allow the music to transport you. Pay attention to any body sensations, images, memories, emotions, or thoughts that come to you as the music carries you into a state of higher consciousness. Allow yourself to fully experience this state and discover what it is like for you. Are you inclined to move your body to express this experience? Would you like to sing? Allow the music to move into and through your body, discovering if there are any places that have a more difficult time receiving it than others. If so, inhale the Sandalwood once again and allow it to assist the music to gently move into this resistant place in your body— as much as feels safe and comfortable. When the music is finished, discover how you feel. What is different from when you first began to listen?

Sandalwood helps you to experience and embody spiritual consciousness in a gentle and safe way.

Aromatic visualization with Sandalwood

Sit quietly. Close your eyes. Take three slow, relaxed, deep breaths. Open your eyes. Put a drop of Sandalwood on a tissue and inhale the aroma through your nose. Pause and inhale again. Visualize a beautiful garden. Imagine that you are floating over this Winter garden, viewing it from above. See this garden as a sacred mandala in which each element is a perfect and precious part that makes up the whole. Is your mandala beautifully complex or elegantly simple? What would be lost if one or another part was not there? Is there anything you might like to add, remove, or change? Take some time to make this mandala appear exactly as you would like it to appear. What does it represent or mean to you? What is its spiritual message for you? Appreciate its wholeness.

Note: A mandala, as it is used here, is any pattern that symbolically represents a microcosm of the universe from the human perspective.

Sandalwood helps you to experience higher consciousness and to understand that many things, including you, contribute to *all that is.*

Aromatic prayer with Sandalwood

Sit quietly. Close your eyes. Take three slow, relaxed, deep breaths. Open your eyes. Put a drop of Sandalwood on a tissue and inhale the aroma through your nose. Pause and inhale again. Pray out loud or internally: "Great Spirit, You of many names and You who cannot be named, help me to become one with You and Your blessed creations. May I grow in Your peace and be at one in Your wisdom. Amen."

Sandalwood helps you to experience a sense of unity and oneness with the Divine.

Elemi

Best essential oil for balancing spiritual and worldly life.

> *The best and safest thing is to keep a*
> *balance in your life, acknowledge the*
> *great powers around us and in us . . .*
> –Euripides

LATIN NAME: *Canarium luzonicum*

EXTRACTED FROM: Resin

PSYCHOLOGICAL PROPERTIES: Uplifts. Promotes a sense of
peace. Relieves stress and nervous exhaustion.

SUBTLE PROPERTIES: Balances spiritual and worldly life.
Promotes a sense of the extraordinary in the ordinary.
Associated with the butterfly in the animal kingdom.

FEBRUARY 15
Aromatic affirmation with Elemi

Sit quietly. Close your eyes. Take three slow, relaxed, deep
breaths. Open your eyes. Put a drop of Elemi on a tissue and
inhale the aroma through your nose. Pause and inhale again.
Say out loud or internally the following affirmation: "I am a
child of both Earth and Spirit. I am in balance and I live in
balance."

Elemi helps you to balance both the physical and spiritual
worlds.

Aromatic emotional self-discovery with Elemi

Sit quietly. Close your eyes. Take three slow, relaxed, deep breaths. Open your eyes. Put a drop of Elemi on a tissue and inhale the aroma through your nose. Pause and inhale again. Ask yourself the following questions and jot down your answers and reflections on a piece of paper.

- What does "balancing spiritual and worldly life" mean to me?
- What aspects of my worldly life support my spirituality?
- Are there aspects of my worldly life that undermine my spirituality?
- What aspects of my spirituality support my worldly life?
- Are there aspects of my spirituality that undermine my worldly life?
- Am I balanced in my spirituality and worldliness? If not, how can I achieve balance?
- How does being balanced in the spiritual and worldly lives benefit me?

Inhale the aroma of Elemi again and intend that you are breathing in a sense of being balanced as both a spiritual and worldly being. Review your answers to the above questions. Reflect and jot down any additional notes.

Elemi helps you to experience balance between your spiritual and worldly lives, and to understand its dynamics in your life.

Aromatic integrating ceremony with Elemi

Sit quietly. Close your eyes. Take three slow, relaxed, deep breaths. Open your eyes. Put a drop of Elemi on a tissue and inhale through your nose. Pause and inhale again. Pour some water into a glass. Hold the glass of water with both hands and intend that it is imbued with light and an invitation to experience the sacredness of ordinary life. As you drink the water, think: "I am filled with light and the ability to experience the ordinary as extraordinary." When you have finished drinking the water, imagine being fully present in body, mind, heart, and spirit, for even the most mundane aspects of your daily life.

Elemi helps you to experience the ordinary as extraordinary.

Aromatic blessing with Elemi

Sit quietly. Close your eyes. Take three slow, relaxed, deep breaths. Open your eyes. Put a drop of Elemi on a tissue and inhale the aroma through your nose. Pause and inhale again. Say out loud or internally: "Bless Spirit as it nourishes all that I do in the physical world. Bless my worldly life in all the ways in which it sustains Spirit. Bless the creative and sacred dance in which Spirit and matter nourish one another, and so, nourish me."

Elemi helps you to experience and understand the ways in which Spirit and matter, when balanced, replenish one another.

Aromatic activity with Elemi

Sit comfortably. Close your eyes. Take three slow, relaxed, deep breaths. Open your eyes. Put a drop of Elemi on a tissue and inhale the aroma through your nose. Pause and inhale again. Rest your hands, palms up, on your lap or your legs. Close your eyes. In your right hand, imagine something that symbolizes your worldly life, such as a stone or a piece of bread. Be present with this item, using your senses of seeing, feeling, hearing, and smelling. In your left hand, imagine something that symbolizes your spiritual life, such as a holy picture, a spiritual icon, or a flower. Experience that item with all your senses in the present moment. Now, slowly and gracefully, lift your hands and gradually bring them together. Notice how your hands join. Are they clasped? Pressed together? Are your fingers straight or curled? Just notice the position they are in. This position represents the integration and balancing of the spiritual and worldly aspects of your life. Whenever you want to experience, remember, or adjust this balance, bring your hands together into this position and intend that the balancing of spiritual and worldly life is occurring.

Elemi helps you to balance your worldly and spiritual lives so that they, together, nurture and sustain you.

Aromatic visualization with Elemi

Sit quietly. Close your eyes. Take three slow, relaxed, deep breaths. Open your eyes. Put a drop of Elemi on a tissue and inhale the aroma through your nose. Pause and inhale again. Visualize a beautiful garden. Observe this Winter garden closely, using all of your senses. What does this garden reveal about your worldly life? What does this garden reveal about your spiritual life? How are these two aspects relating to one another in this garden? Do their messages balance? Are they at odds with each other in any way? Is there anything that you would like to change in order to bring greater balance? Acknowledge and appreciate the graceful and sacred way in which Spirit and matter manifest here. Spend some time examining this garden from the perspective of both the physical and spiritual dimensions.

Elemi helps you to experience how matter and Spirit relate to one another.

Aromatic prayer with Elemi

Sit quietly. Close your eyes. Take three slow, relaxed, deep breaths. Open your eyes. Put a drop of Elemi on a tissue and inhale the aroma through your nose. Pause and inhale again. Pray out loud or internally: "Dear God, You who creates the beauty in this material world, bless and heal me. Dear God, You who guides me on my spiritual path, bless and heal me. May I balance these worlds in the oneness of You. Amen."

Elemi helps you to experience balance in your life as part of the oneness of the Divine.

Frankincense

Best essential oil for spiritual wisdom. Embodies the spirit of Winter.

> *Pain and foolishness lead*
> *to great bliss and complete knowledge,*
> *for Eternal Wisdom created nothing*
> *under the sun in vain.*
> –Kahlil Gibran

LATIN NAME: *Boswellia carterii*

EXTRACTED FROM: Resin

PSYCHOLOGICAL PROPERTIES: Calms the mind. Relieves stress, anxiety, and nervous tension.

SUBTLE PROPERTIES: Promotes and supports spiritual wisdom. Associated with the archangel Raziel in the angelic realm and the owl in the animal kingdom.

FEBRUARY 22
Aromatic affirmation with Frankincense

Sit quietly. Close your eyes. Take three slow, relaxed, deep breaths. Open your eyes. Put a drop of Frankincense on a tissue and inhale the aroma through your nose. Pause and inhale again. Say out loud or internally the following affirmation: "Spiritual wisdom fills my body, mind, heart, and spirit. This is my true nature."

Frankincense helps you to experience and embody spiritual wisdom.

Aromatic emotional self-discovery with Frankincense

Sit quietly. Close your eyes. Take three slow, relaxed, deep breaths. Open your eyes. Put a drop of Frankincense on a tissue and inhale the aroma through your nose. Pause and inhale again. Ask yourself the following questions and jot down your answers and reflections on a piece of paper.

⤚ What does "spiritual wisdom" mean to me?

⤚ What are the gifts of spiritual wisdom?

⤚ What are the challenges of spiritual wisdom?

⤚ What promotes spiritual wisdom for me?

⤚ What hinders spiritual wisdom for me?

⤚ How do I benefit from spiritual wisdom?

Inhale the aroma of Frankincense again and intend that you are breathing in spiritual wisdom. Review your answers to the above questions. Reflect and jot down any additional notes.

Frankincense helps you to experience and strengthen spiritual wisdom and to understand its dynamics in your life.

Aromatic manifesting ceremony with Frankincense

Sit quietly. Close your eyes. Take three slow, relaxed, deep breaths. Open your eyes. Find or create an object that represents "spiritual wisdom" for you, such as a lit candle or a picture of someone you honor as a wise being. Set it in front of you. Put a drop of Frankincense on a tissue and inhale the aroma through your nose. Pause and inhale again. Hold your hands over or around the object as you send the intention of spiritual wisdom into the object. From now on, whenever you see, touch, or remember this object, the sense of spiritual wisdom will be with you in body, mind, heart, and spirit. If you choose, place the object in a special place as a reminder.

Frankincense helps you to experience spiritual wisdom and to receive the support you need on your spiritual journey.

Aromatic blessing with Frankincense

Sit quietly. Close your eyes. Take three slow, relaxed, deep breaths. Open your eyes. Put a drop of Frankincense on a tissue and inhale the aroma through your nose. Pause and inhale again. Say out loud or internally the following blessing: "Bless each step I take toward spiritual wisdom. Bless each experience that assists me to grow stronger in spiritual wisdom. Bless the teachers, the helpers, and the many lessons that guide me on this journey."

Frankincense helps you to experience spiritual wisdom and to bless all that contributes to it.

Aromatic activity with Frankincense

Sit quietly. Close your eyes. Take three slow, relaxed, deep breaths. Open your eyes. Put a drop of Frankincense on a tissue and inhale the aroma through your nose. Pause and inhale again. Sit quietly, your spine straight and your body relaxed. Begin to observe your breath. Whenever you notice a thought, simple name it "thought," and come back to your breath. If you notice a feeling, gently name it for its attributes, such as anger, fear, or joy, and then come back to your breath. Do the same with any sensation—identify and name it, such as pain, tension, or warmth—and then come back to your breath. Without judgment, simply witness the activity of your mind, emotions, and senses, and then gently come back to your breath. Do this activity for ten minutes and notice how you feel at the end of it.

Frankincense helps to gently develop the spiritual wisdom and practice of nonjudgment.

FEBRUARY 27
Aromatic visualization with Frankincense

Sit quietly. Close your eyes. Take three slow, relaxed, deep breaths. Open your eyes. Put a drop of Frankincense on a tissue and inhale the aroma through your nose. Pause and inhale again. Visualize a beautiful garden. Walk slowly through this Winter garden, breathing deeply, and be aware of the sunlight here that surrounds you and everything in the garden. How would you describe this light? How does it appear and feel to you? Now, imagine that this light represents spiritual wisdom. If it were to speak to you, what would it say? If it were to create an image for you, what would it be? If it had something to teach you, what would the lesson be? Now imagine yourself being embraced by this light and be open to receiving its gifts.

Frankincense helps you to experience and explore the inner light of spiritual wisdom.

Aromatic prayer with Frankincense

Sit quietly. Close your eyes. Take three slow, relaxed, deep breaths. Open your eyes. Put a drop of Frankincense on a tissue and inhale the aroma through your nose. Pause and inhale again. Pray out loud or internally: "Divine One, help me to embrace Your light of spiritual wisdom. Help me to see it in the brightness and in the darkness. May it shine within me, around me, and through me. Amen."

Frankincense helps you to experience the divine light of spiritual wisdom.

End-of-the-Month Day

FEBRUARY 29

Aromatic ceremony to honor your accomplishments this Winter

Choose one of your favorite essential oils among the Winter essential oils: Benzoin, Vetiver, Vanilla, Oakmoss, Neroli, Spikenard, Myrrh, Rosewood, Immortelle, Cedarwood, Sandalwood, Elemi, and Frankincense. Sit quietly. Close your eyes. Take three slow, relaxed, deep breaths. Open your eyes. Put a drop of your chosen oil on a tissue and inhale the aroma through your nose. Pause and inhale again. Reflect back upon the past Winter season and identify your accomplishments. Don't be modest. Notice each and every goal you have accomplished, from the small to the large. Inhale your oil once again, and take a large step forward. As you do, say out loud or internally, "I have accomplished _____ this Winter." Inhale your oil again, and take another step, saying out loud or internally, "I have also accomplished _____ in these last few months." With one more step and one final inhalation, say out loud or internally, "I want to be sure I acknowledge accomplishing _____." Now turn around and visualize looking back at yourself prior to taking these three steps. Notice how, in only a few minutes, something has changed within you simply through the process of acknowledging what you have accomplished. Now ask yourself what you might like to do to celebrate what you have accomplished. This could be watching a favorite old movie, reading a new inspirational book, or visiting a beautiful church. You may wish to celebrate with a friend. Think of something that would please you and make a commitment to do this for yourself now, to honor your accomplishments this Winter.

Note: February 29 comes only every four years. In order to honor your accomplishments for the Winter in the years in which February has only twenty-eight days, do this exercise in addition to the exercise for February 28.

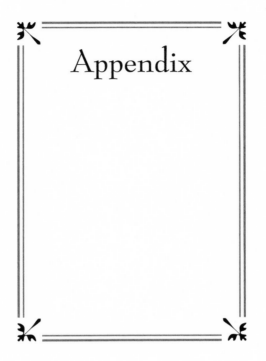

Appendix

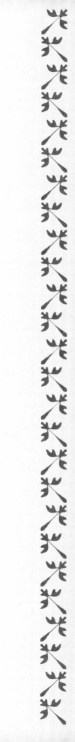

Appendix I
Best Essential Oil for ...

Every essential oil profiled in *Daily Aromatherapy* is designated as an oil that is "best for" a particular quality. That information is collected here for easy reference.

Spring is the season of the soul that signals optimism and hope. It is a time to clear away and release what no longer serves you—physically, mentally, emotionally, and spiritually—so that you can experience rebirth, inspiration, and renewed creativity. It is a time for new beginnings, new experiences, new relationships, and new perspectives on existing relationships. Spring is the season that represents the feminine, and also the childhood stage of your life.

March
March is the first Spring month. Its theme is to clear away, cleanse, and release, so that you can move forward, unburdened, toward your aspirations, dreams, hopes, desires, goals, and Highest Self.

- Lemongrass: Best oil to clear and cleanse.
- Bay St. Thomas: Best oil for releasing fear.

- Grapefruit: Best oil to release negative emotions.
- Juniper Berry: Best oil for protecting against negativity and negative influences.

April

April is the second Spring month. It is the time to open your heart to the joy of being alive. It is the time to experience hope and optimism for the present and the future.

- Orange: Best oil for joy.
- Mandarin: Best oil for optimism.
- Petitgrain: Best oil for harmonious relationships.
- Bergamot: Best oil for hope.

May

May is the third and last Spring month. It is a time to be receptive to, as well as initiate, new beginnings. It is a time of rebirth and inspiration, and for creative expression to find fertile soil.

- Geranium: Best oil to support the feminine.
- Coriander: Best oil for creativity.
- Nutmeg: Best oil to support new beginnings.
- Eucalyptus: Best oil for inspiration.
- Mimosa: Best oil for renewal.

Summer is the season of the soul that signals manifestation and full expression—the foundation for which is mental clarity, concentration, and focus. Your body, mind, heart, and spirit are energized and motivated, moving your thoughts into action. Fortitude, courage, and confidence help to bring your heart and soul's desire to fruition. Summer is the season that symbolizes the masculine and represents the young-adult stage of your life.

June

June is the first Summer month. It is a time to gain clarity, and to concentrate and focus on what you want to manifest in the world. This lays a strong foundation for achieving your aspirations.

- ↞ Rosemary: Best oil for mental clarity.
- ↞ Basil: Best oil for concentration.
- ↞ Lemon: Best oil for objectivity.
- ↞ Peppermint: Best oil for mental energy.

July

July is the second Summer month. It is the time to exert and demonstrate your energy and willpower to achieve your aspirations with the support of unwavering confidence and courage.

- Pine: Best oil for willpower.
- Cinnamon: Best oil for confidence.
- Thyme: Best oil to support the masculine.
- Tea Tree: Best oil for energizing on all levels.
- German Chamomile: Best oil for truthful expression.

August

August is the last Summer month. It is the time for the manifestation and achievement of your dreams and desires via personal motivation, passion, and perseverance.

- Clove: Best oil for motivation.
- Ginger: Best oil for manifesting.
- Ylang Ylang: Best oil for passion and enthusiasm.
- Fennel: Best oil for perseverance.

Autumn is the season of the soul that signals a time to reflect on your life and assess the health and well-being of your body, mind, heart, and spirit. It is a time for insights and using good judgment regarding your relationships, how you take care of yourself, how you spend your time, and what you have accomplished. Forgiving and accepting your shortcomings, as well as the shortcomings of others, help you

pave the way to a peaceful heart. It is also a time to acknowledge and be grateful for the many blessings in your life, and
to be generous of spirit. In all of this, healing takes place.
Autumn represents the mid-life stage of your life.

September

September is the first Autumn month. It is a time for self-
reflection and understanding, the use of good judgment, and
the development of insight, awareness, and intuition.

> ⤙ Spruce: Best oil for self-reflection.
>
> ⤙ Fir: Best oil for self-understanding.
>
> ⤙ Bay Laurel: Best oil for using good judgment.
>
> ⤙ Clary Sage: Best oil for intuition.

October

October is the second Autumn month. It is a time for moving forward from self-reflection and understanding to self-
acceptance, forgiveness, and healing.

> ⤙ Palmarosa: Best oil for self-acceptance.
>
> ⤙ Roman Chamomile: Best oil for forgiveness.
>
> ⤙ Marjoram: Best oil for healing grief.
>
> ⤙ Lavender: Best oil for healing on all levels.
>
> ⤙ Champaca: Best oil for receptivity to spiritual
> guidance.

November

November is the last Autumn month. It is a time to reflect on the many blessings in your life and to have an attitude of gratitude and generosity. It is a time for personal growth, transformation, and the development of compassion.

- Jasmine: Best oil for gratitude.
- Cardamom: Best oil for generosity.
- Cypress: Best oil for personal growth.
- Rose: Best oil for compassion and unconditional love.

Winter is the season of the soul that signals rest. It is a time to feel comfortable, safe, and secure—in body, mind, heart, and spirit. A sense of being *home* embraces you. There is an awareness of wholeness, satisfaction, and abundance. It is a time of peace and trust, and in that, there is restoration and rejuvenation. It is a time when increasing wisdom can lead the way to contemplative spirituality. Winter is the season that represents the senior stage of your life.

December

December is the first Winter month. It is a time to feel comfortable, warm, safe, and secure. This well-grounded state helps you to build the inner strength that supports the progression to higher states of consciousness.

⤙ Benzoin: Best oil for comfort.

⤙ Vetiver: Best oil for feeling safe.

⤙ Vanilla: Best oil for deep, nurturing connection to Mother Earth.

⤙ Oakmoss: Best oil for a sense of abundance.

January

January is the second Winter month. It is a time to rest and be at peace, allowing your spirit to rejuvenate and restore. It is the time to trust, surrender, and be still.

⤙ Neroli: Best oil for a sense of peace.

⤙ Spikenard: Best oil for a sense of trust.

⤙ Myrrh: Best oil to understand the spiritual perspective of emotional challenges.

⤙ Rosewood: Best oil for spiritual opening and growth.

⤙ Immortelle: Best oil for spiritual strength.

February

February is the last Winter month. It is the time to rest in wisdom and enlightenment. You shall live balanced in the realm of the physical world and the spiritual world. Your Higher Self—the part of you that is evolved and connected to the Divine—experiences a sense of oneness as you embrace true spirituality.

- Cedarwood: Best oil for a direct connection with the Divine.
- Sandalwood: Best oil for a sense of oneness.
- Elemi: Best oil for balancing spiritual and worldly life.
- Frankincense: Best oil for spiritual wisdom.

Appendix II
Alternate and Additional Best Essential Oils

Every essential oil has a variety of properties. Many essential oils share similar properties with other essential oils—for example, Peppermint, Rosemary, and Eucalyptus are all energizing oils. The information below is organized by season. Italics indicate the oil chosen and highlighted in the book as the best choice for that season's particular theme. As an example, for clearing and cleansing, *Lemongrass* is the best choice. However, in some cases, you may not care for the aroma of the designated essential oil, or you may not have it. You may want to use a different oil. This list serves as a reference to choose a different oil with similar properties.

Spring is the season of the soul that signals optimism and hope. It is a time to clear away and release what no longer serves you—physically, mentally, emotionally, and spiritually—so that you can experience rebirth, inspiration, and renewed creativity. It is a time for new beginnings, new experiences, new relationships, and new perspectives on existing relationships. Spring is the season that represents the feminine, and also the childhood stage of your life.

- Childhood: Mandarin, Orange, Nutmeg, Mimosa
- Clearing and Cleansing (for new beginnings): *Lemongrass,* Eucalyptus, Juniper Berry, Rosemary
- Creativity: *Coriander,* Clary Sage, Jasmine
- Feminine: *Geranium,* Jasmine, Neroli
- Hope: *Bergamot,* Orange, Spikenard
- Inspiration: *Eucalyptus,* Clary Sage, Jasmine, Fir
- Joy: *Orange,* Mandarin, Neroli
- Negativity, dispel: Juniper Berry, Orange, Lemon, Bergamot, Lemongrass, Grapefruit
- Negativity, protection from: *Juniper Berry,* Fennel
- New beginnings (relationships, experiences): *Nutmeg,* Lavender, Ylang Ylang
- Optimism: *Mandarin,* Rose, Orange, Neroli, Bergamot, Mimosa
- Positivity: Orange, Bergamot, Lemon, Cedarwood
- Rebirth: Lavender, Cypress, Rose
- Relationships (harmonious): *Petitgrain,* Jasmine, Geranium, Ylang Ylang, Rose
- Releasing, anger: Ylang Ylang, Benzoin
- Releasing, fear: *Bay St. Thomas,* Frankincense, Geranium
- Releasing, frustration: Grapefruit, Marjoram, Lavender

- ⤙ Releasing, grief: Bergamot, Roman Chamomile
- ⤙ Releasing, negative emotions: *Grapefruit,* Juniper Berry
- ⤙ Renewal: *Mimosa,* Orange, Mandarin

Summer is the season of the soul that signals manifestation and full expression—the foundation for which is mental clarity, concentration, and focus. Your body, mind, heart, and spirit are energized and motivated, moving your thoughts into action. Fortitude, courage, and confidence help to bring your heart and soul's desire to fruition. Summer is the season that symbolizes the masculine and represents the young-adult stage of your life.

- ⤙ Activity: Cinnamon, Peppermint, Rosemary, Eucalyptus, Ginger
- ⤙ Alertness: Basil, Lemongrass, Rosemary, Peppermint
- ⤙ Concentration: *Basil,* Lemongrass, Rosemary
- ⤙ Confidence: *Cinnamon,* Cedarwood, Tea Tree, Thyme
- ⤙ Courage: Thyme, Frankincense, Ginger
- ⤙ Emotional fortitude: Geranium, Ylang Ylang, Marjoram, Thyme
- ⤙ Energy: *Tea Tree,* Pine, Rosemary, Peppermint

- Enjoyment: Jasmine, Orange, Sandalwood, Ylang Ylang, Rose, Cardamom
- Enthusiasm: *Ylang Ylang,* Orange, Cardamom, Jasmine
- Focus: Basil, Benzoin, Rosemary, Lemon
- Heart's desire: Lavender, Rose, Sandalwood, Ylang Ylang, Mimosa
- Manifesting: *Ginger,* Pine, Nutmeg, Basil, Rosemary
- Masculine: *Thyme,* Cedarwood
- Mental clarity: *Rosemary,* Geranium, Lemon
- Mental energy: *Peppermint,* Eucalyptus, Thyme
- Motivation: *Clove,* Mandarin, Tea Tree, Rosemary
- Objectivity: *Lemon,* Basil, Rosemary
- Passion: *Ylang Ylang,* Jasmine, Sandalwood, Cardamom
- Perseverance: *Fennel,* Lemon, Tea Tree
- Play: Orange, Mandarin
- Truthful expression: *German Chamomile*
- Willpower: *Pine,* Rosemary, Cedarwood, Tea Tree, Thyme
- Young adult: Thyme, Tea Tree, Cinnamon, Ginger, Ylang Ylang

Autumn is the season of the soul that signals a time to reflect on your life and assess the health and well-being of your body, mind, heart, and spirit. It is a time for insights and using good judgment regarding your relationships, how you take care of yourself, how you spend your time, and what you have accomplished. Forgiving and accepting your shortcomings, as well as the shortcomings of others, help you pave the way to a peaceful heart. It is also a time to acknowledge and be grateful for the many blessings in your life, and to be generous of spirit. In all of this, healing takes place. Autumn represents the mid-life stage of your life.

- Awareness: Sandalwood, Lavender, Oakmoss, Elemi, Frankincense
- Compassion: *Rose,* Bergamot, Spikenard
- Forgiveness: *Roman Chamomile,* Rose, Frankincense
- Friendship, true: Rose, Sandalwood, Cardamom
- Generosity: *Cardamom,* Geranium, Bergamot
- Good judgment/Discernment: *Bay Laurel,* Basil
- Gratitude: *Jasmine,* Ginger
- Guidance, spiritual: *Champaca,* Sandalwood, Frankincense, Cedarwood
- Healing, all levels (body, mind, spirit): *Lavender,* Palmarosa, Rose

- Healing, grief: *Marjoram,* Bergamot, Rose
- Insight: Lemon, Rosemary, Peppermint, Bay Laurel
- Intuition: *Clary Sage,* Bay Laurel, Fir, Spruce
- Love, promotes: Bergamot, Rose
- Love, unconditional: *Rose,* Sandalwood
- Mid-life: Cypress, Lavender, Palmarosa, Jasmine
- Personal growth: *Cypress,* Lavender, Frankincense
- Self-acceptance: *Palmarosa,* Bergamot
- Self-reflection: *Spruce,* Sandalwood, Cedarwood
- Self-understanding: *Fir,* Rosemary, Lemon
- Sharing: Cardamom, Geranium, Rose
- Teaching (passing on gained knowledge): Cardamom, Vetiver, German Chamomile

Winter is the season of the soul that signals rest. It is a time to feel comfortable, safe, and secure—in body, mind, heart, and spirit. A sense of being *home* embraces you. There is an awareness of wholeness, satisfaction, and abundance. It is a time of peace and trust, and in that, there is restoration and rejuvenation. It is a time when increasing wisdom can lead the way to contemplative spirituality. Winter is the season that represents the senior stage of your life.

- Abundance: *Oakmoss,* Nutmeg, Ginger
- Comfort: *Benzoin,* Bergamot, Rose, Vanilla, Sandalwood
- Divine, devotion to: Sandalwood, Rose, Myrrh, Frankincense
- Divine, direct connection to: *Cedarwood,* Elemi, Frankincense
- Faith: *Spikenard,* Myrrh, Rosemary
- Grounding: Oakmoss, Cedarwood, Vetiver, Vanilla
- Harmony: Lavender, Vetiver, Rose, Geranium, Petitgrain
- Higher Self: Cedarwood, Elemi, Sandalwood, Frankincense, Myrrh
- Home: Vetiver, Vanilla, Coriander, Benzoin
- Mother Earth (connection to): *Vanilla,* Oakmoss, Vetiver
- Mysticism: Elemi, Sandalwood, Cedarwood, Frankincense, Rosewood
- Oneness: *Sandalwood,* Frankincense, Cedarwood, Elemi
- Peace: *Neroli,* Rose, Chamomile, Lavender
- Prosperity: *Oakmoss,* Ginger
- Rejuvenation: Lemon, Orange, Bergamot, Rosemary
- Rest: Roman Chamomile, Lavender, Rose

- Restoration: Juniper Berry, Spruce, Pine
- Safe (feeling): *Vetiver,* Benzoin, Vanilla, Frankincense
- Security: Oakmoss, Ginger, Myrrh
- Senior years: Myrrh, Cypress, Frankincense, Roman Chamomile
- Spiritual strength: *Immortelle*
- Spiritual wisdom: *Frankincense,* Sandalwood
- Spirituality, balance (with worldly life): *Elemi,* Lavender
- Spirituality, growth (preparing for): *Rosewood,* Jasmine
- Spirituality, perspective of emotional challenges: *Myrrh,* Rose
- Trust: *Spikenard,* Mandarin, Myrrh
- Wholeness: Sandalwood, Frankincense, Lavender, Elemi
- Wisdom: *Frankincense,* Sandalwood, Cedarwood

Appendix III
Essential Oils for Difficult Mental and Emotional Issues

Following is a list of difficult mental and emotional issues and the essential oils that may be helpful to affect them in a positive way.

- ⤙ Abandonment: Rose, Bergamot, Frankincense
- ⤙ Absentmindedness: Rosemary, Lemon, Peppermint, Basil, Cedarwood, Lemongrass
- ⤙ Addiction: Bergamot, Eucalyptus, Spearmint
- ⤙ Anger: Roman Chamomile, Ylang Ylang, Grapefruit, Bergamot, Frankincense
- ⤙ Anxiety: Neroli, Roman Chamomile, Frankincense, Lavender, Sandalwood
- ⤙ Apathy: Orange, Mandarin, Rosemary, Thyme, Myrrh, Lemon, Geranium
- ⤙ Betrayal: Roman Chamomile, Bergamot, Juniper Berry, Sandalwood
- ⤙ Bitterness: Orange, Roman Chamomile, Rose, Bergamot, Frankincense, Lemon, Vetiver
- ⤙ Boredom: Rosemary, Orange, Thyme
- ⤙ Burden: Eucalyptus, Pine, Frankincense, Mandarin, Orange, Lemon

- Burnout: Mimosa, Eucalyptus, Frankincense, Pine, Lavender
- Compulsiveness: Clary Sage, Spearmint, Grapefruit
- Confusion: Rosemary, Lemon, Peppermint, Basil, Geranium
- Cornered: Eucalyptus, Lemongrass, Lemon, Bay St. Thomas, Grapefruit, Nutmeg
- Critical: Palmarosa, Roman Chamomile, Lavender, Rosewood, Cedarwood, Sandalwood
- Cynical: Sandalwood, Spikenard, Rose, Frankincense, Neroli, Mandarin
- Defeated: Orange, Vetiver, Bergamot, Lemon, Pine, Thyme, Ginger
- Depression: Orange, Geranium, Ylang Ylang, Bergamot, Clary Sage, Jasmine, Mandarin
- Desperation: Roman Chamomile, Lavender, Vetiver
- Despondency: Orange, Bergamot, Clary Sage, Mandarin, Cedarwood, Juniper Berry
- Devastation: Rose, Bergamot, Frankincense, Lavender
- Disappointment: Marjoram, Lavender, Myrrh
- Discouragement: Orange, Lemon, Pine, Eucalyptus, Juniper Berry

- Disgust: Lemon, Tea Tree, Eucalyptus, Roman Chamomile, Pine
- Disorientation: Rosemary, Peppermint, Lemongrass, Tea Tree
- Doubt: Spikenard, Tea Tree, Peppermint
- Dread: Rose, Bergamot, Lavender, Bay St. Thomas, Grapefruit, Palmarosa
- Embarrassment: Peppermint, Jasmine, Tea Tree, Cedarwood, Vetiver
- Emptiness: Sandalwood, Marjoram, Petitgrain, Mandarin, Neroli
- Exhaustion (emotional): Frankincense, Geranium, Orange, Mimosa, Pine, Lavender
- Fatigue: Rosemary, Peppermint, Pine, Tea Tree, Lemongrass
- Fear: Ylang Ylang, Spikenard, Marjoram, Bay St. Thomas, Lavender, Sandalwood, Lemon
- Frustration: Ylang Ylang, Frankincense, Rose, German Chamomile
- Grief: Marjoram, Rose, Bergamot, Frankincense, Neroli, Cypress
- Guilt: Ylang Ylang, Rose, Frankincense, Juniper Berry
- Heartbroken: Rose, Marjoram, Bergamot, Neroli
- Heartsick: Rose, Bergamot, Benzoin

- Helpless: Thyme, Ginger, Cinnamon, Tea Tree, Peppermint
- Hopeless: Bergamot, Orange, Mandarin, Spikenard
- Humiliation: Peppermint, Petitgrain, Vetiver
- Hurt: Rose, Lavender, Palmarosa
- Hyperactivity: Clary Sage, Roman Chamomile, Lavender, Ylang Ylang
- Impatience: Roman Chamomile, Lavender, Rose, Ylang Ylang
- Impulsiveness: Roman Chamomile, Frankincense, Sandalwood, Vetiver
- Inadequacy: Cinnamon, Thyme, Pine, Tea Tree, Ginger, Ylang Ylang, Cedarwood
- Indecisiveness: Rosemary, Lemon, Basil, Clove
- Indignant: Ylang Ylang, Roman Chamomile
- Insecurity: Vetiver, Vanilla, Frankincense, Ylang Ylang, Bergamot, Peppermint
- Irritability: Roman Chamomile, Lavender, Ylang Ylang, Sandalwood
- Jealousy: Ylang Ylang, Clary Sage, Rose, Frankincense, Cypress, Petitgrain, Mandarin
- Judgmental: Bergamot, Rose, Roman Chamomile, Frankincense, Ylang Ylang
- Laziness: Rosemary, Peppermint, Lemon, Pine, Tea Tree, Cypress

- Lethargy: Rosemary, Peppermint, Pine, Ginger, Lemon
- Loneliness: Marjoram, Petitgrain, Sandalwood
- Loss: Marjoram, Bergamot, Rose
- Melancholy: Orange, Bergamot, Rose, Ylang Ylang
- Moodiness: Lavender, Geranium, Eucalyptus
- Nightmares: Lavender, Frankincense
- Obsessive: Sandalwood, Clary Sage
- Obstinate: Orange, Rosewood, Ylang Ylang
- Offended: Rose, Bergamot, Ylang Ylang, Bergamot, Jasmine, Juniper Berry
- Outrage: Roman Chamomile, Ylang Ylang, Grapefruit, Lavender, Sandalwood, Frankincense
- Overwhelm: Peppermint, Rosemary, Pine, Tea Tree, Frankincense, Rosewood
- Paranoid: Lavender, Frankincense, Sandalwood
- Persecution: Oakmoss, Vetiver, Myrrh
- Pressure: Eucalyptus, Lemongrass, Ginger, Tea Tree, Rosemary, Juniper Berry
- Procrastination: Sandalwood, Lemon, Thyme, Rosemary, Peppermint
- Rage: Roman Chamomile, Ylang Ylang, Frankincense, Lemon
- Rejection: Rose, Bergamot, Roman Chamomile

- Resentfulness: Sandalwood, Ylang Ylang, Clary Sage, Lemon
- Restlessness: Lavender, Neroli, Roman Chamomile, Sandalwood, Frankincense
- Rigidity: Geranium, Lavender, Sandalwood, Frankincense, Neroli
- Sadness: Orange, Mandarin, Jasmine, Rose, Ylang Ylang
- Self-consciousness: Ylang Ylang, Pine, Juniper Berry
- Selfishness: Sandalwood, Frankincense, Rose, Sandalwood, Orange, Rose
- Sensitivity: Mimosa, Sandalwood, Ylang Ylang
- Shameful: Rosemary, Rose, Ylang Ylang
- Shattered: Orange, Bergamot, Rose, Frankincense, Tea Tree, Vetiver, Ylang Ylang
- Shock: Tea Tree, Ylang Ylang, Frankincense, Sandalwood, Bergamot, Clary Sage
- Shyness: Ylang Ylang, Petitgrain, Thyme, Lavender
- Stress (general): Roman Chamomile, Lavender, Clary Sage, Ylang Ylang, Frankincense
- Stubbornness: Mandarin, Orange
- Suspicious: Ylang Ylang, Rose, Sandalwood, Orange, Spikenard

- Tiredness: Rosemary, Peppermint, Tea Tree, Pine, Juniper Berry, Lemongrass
- Trapped: Eucalyptus, Lemongrass, Bay St. Thomas, Grapefruit, Nutmeg, Sandalwood
- Trauma: Rose, Roman Chamomile, Tea Tree, Ylang Ylang
- Unforgiving: Roman Chamomile, Palmarosa, Sandalwood, Frankincense, Spikenard, Bergamot
- Untrusting: Spikenard, Vetiver, Oakmoss, Myrrh
- Vulnerability: Mimosa, Juniper Berry, Vetiver, Benzoin
- Withdrawn: Marjoram, Orange, Neroli, Thyme, Rosemary
- Worn out: Mimosa, Frankincense, Pine, Tea Tree, Orange, Lemon
- Worry: Roman Chamomile, Lavender, Sandalwood, Frankincense, Cedarwood

Appendix IV

Essential Oils and Associated Archangels

Aromas have long been used in a spiritual context as an offering to the heavens, to connect with the Divine, and to assist with healing, prayer, and meditation. This association is deeply rooted in tradition—incense is burned in Christian churches and Buddhist temples, Native Americans use fragrant herbs in their sweat lodges to facilitate a spiritual connection, and Tibetans burn bundles of Juniper to accompany their prayers. Different aromas are favored by different cultures and spiritual practices.

The premier aromas associated with angels are Rose and Jasmine. Rose is considered to be the aroma *of* angels—the aroma being detected upon their arrival and their departure. Jasmine is an aroma *favored* by angels, and smelling or wearing it helps to bring you closer to the angelic realm.

Rose and Jasmine are the best-known angelic aromas but there are others, and there are those that associate particularly well with the archangels, as listed below. The meaning of the individual archangel's name is in quotes. If you would like to learn more about the archangels, our favorite reference book is *Archangels and Ascended Masters* (2004) by Doreen Virtue.

To use the associated essential oils, sit quietly and close your eyes. Take three slow, relaxed, deep breaths. Open your eyes. Put a drop of the chosen essential oil on a tissue and inhale the aroma through your nose. Pause and inhale again. Close your eyes. With the intent of calling the associated archangel to be at your side, inhale the aroma again. Ask that they be with you and call them by name, either out loud or internally. Visualize and feel their presence. Dialogue with them, if you like, or simply sit with them. When you are finished, thank them.

∾ Essential Oils and the Archangels ↙

Archangel Ariel — "Lioness of God"

KEYWORD: Courage

ASSOCIATIONS: Courage, confidence, manifestation, protection of nature, support for healers, divine magic, life's mission, prosperity.

BEST ESSENTIAL OIL:

- ⊷ Ginger: Promotes courage, confidence, and prosperity. Helps to manifest your heart's desire.

ADDITIONAL ESSENTIAL OILS:

- ⊷ Cinnamon: Promotes confidence and courage.
- ⊷ Nutmeg: Supports new beginnings and prosperity.

⊷ Rosemary: Supports manifesting your desires.

⊷ Rose: Promotes unconditional love.

Archangel Azrael — "Whom God Helps"

KEYWORD: Comfort

ASSOCIATIONS: Comfort, especially for those crossing over to heaven, support for those grieving for loss of loved ones, quiet strength, support for helpers.

BEST ESSENTIAL OIL:

Sandalwood: Comforts. Provides emotional support and quiet strength.

ADDITIONAL ESSENTIAL OILS:

⊷ Rose: Provides comfort. Promotes love and heals the wounds of the heart. Connects with the angels.

⊷ Cypress: Provides support during times of transition. Strengthens and comforts.

⊷ Bergamot: Eases grief.

Archangel Chamuel — "He Who Sees God"

KEYWORD: Clear sight

ASSOCIATIONS: "See" clearly, third eye, meaningful relationships and work, personal and global peace, protection against negativity, love of life.

BEST ESSENTIAL OIL:

⊷ Yarrow: Promotes visions and psychic awareness. Promotes love and harmony.

ADDITIONAL ESSENTIAL OILS:

- ⤙ Bergamot: Promotes positive energy and love.
- ⤙ German Chamomile: Promotes peace, patience, and forgiveness.
- ⤙ Vetiver: Protects.
- ⤙ Clary Sage: Strengthens the "inner eye" to "see" more clearly.
- ⤙ Rosemary: Promotes healthy boundaries in relationships.

Archangel Gabriel — "God Is My Strength"

KEYWORD: Strength

ASSOCIATIONS: Strength, action, power, "the messenger," communication, inspiration for creative expression, parenthood, children and inner child.

BEST ESSENTIAL OIL:

- ⤙ Rosemary: Strengthens and centers. Promotes action.

ADDITIONAL ESSENTIAL OILS:

- ⤙ Rosewood: Nurtures the inner child. Promotes creative expression.
- ⤙ Bay Laurel: Opens and encourages communication and creative expression.
- ⤙ German Chamomile: Promotes truthful communication.
- ⤙ Rose: Nurtures and comforts.

- ⤙ Coriander: Promotes creative expression and spontaneity.
- ⤙ Mandarin: Promotes childlike exuberance and joy.

Archangel Haniel — "Grace of God"

KEYWORD: Moon energy

ASSOCIATIONS: Moon energy, highest potential, sensitivity, psychic abilities, patience, harmony, mystical, clairvoyance, natural healing remedies, hidden talents.

BEST ESSENTIAL OIL:

- ⤙ German Chamomile: Increases intuition and psychic abilities. Promotes patience.

ADDITIONAL ESSENTIAL OILS:

- ⤙ Jasmine: Helps in understanding deeper truths. Promotes intuition, beauty, and passion.
- ⤙ Rose: Promotes appreciation of beauty. Promotes harmony and grace.
- ⤙ Sandalwood: Promotes and supports higher consciousness.
- ⤙ Juniper Berry: Promotes high ideals.

Archangel Jeremiel — "Mercy of God"

KEYWORD: Prophecy

ASSOCIATIONS: Prophetic dreams and visions, life review, releases old patterns, positive changes, gratitude, love, core archangel.

-+ Clary Sage: Promotes visions and dreams. Promotes forgiveness. Strengthens the "inner eye." Promotes a state of euphoria.

ADDITIONAL ESSENTIAL OILS:

-+ Jasmine: Promotes gratitude.

-+ Spruce: Promotes self-reflection and objectivity.

-+ Grapefruit: Releases negative emotions and patterns. Clears and cleanses.

-+ Bergamot: Promotes self-love, self-acceptance, and positivity.

-+ Rose: Promotes love of self and others.

Archangel Jophiel — "Beauty of God"

KEYWORD: Beauty

ASSOCIATIONS: Art and beauty, beauty in everything and everyone, beautiful thoughts, slowing down to enjoy life, inspiration for artistic endeavors, fun.

BEST ESSENTIAL OIL:

-+ Jasmine: Promotes love of beauty, the arts, creativity, artistic development, and sensuality. Opens the heart. Enhances intuition. Inspires.

ADDITIONAL ESSENTIAL OILS:

-+ Rose: Promotes love of beauty and patience. Helps us to slow down.

- Orange: Uplifts and promotes positive energy.
- Coriander: Promotes creative expression and spontaneity.
- Roman Chamomile: Promotes patience. Helps us to slow down.

Archangel Metatron — (meaning of name unclear)

KEYWORD: Motivation

ASSOCIATIONS: Motivation, mental energy, focus, fortitude, fiery strength, record keeper, organization, helps special children, youngest archangel, one of only two archangels who have been mortal, twin to Sandalphon.

BEST ESSENTIAL OIL:

- Black Pepper: Promotes strength, fortitude, and motivation.

ADDITIONAL ESSENTIAL OILS:

- Clove: Promotes motivation.
- Peppermint: Increases mental energy, clarity, and focus. Increases concentration.
- Myrrh: Bridges upper and lower energy centers and heaven and earth.
- Mandarin: Helps us to connect with our inner child. Promotes childlike joy.
- Juniper Berry: Clears and cleanses. Promotes intuition.

Archangel Michael — "He Who Is Like God"

KEYWORD: Cast out fear

ASSOCIATIONS: Release of fear, protection, fiery energy, action, motivation, archangel leader, oversee lightworkers, guidance for life purpose or career, self-esteem, confidence.

BEST ESSENTIAL OIL:

- ⤙ Thyme: Promotes courage, power, strength, confidence, and action.

ADDITIONAL ESSENTIAL OILS:

- ⤙ Rose: Promotes divine love. Helps to dissipate fear.
- ⤙ Rosemary: Inspires faith. Promotes action.
- ⤙ Cinnamon: Promotes courage, confidence, strength, fiery energy, and action.
- ⤙ Juniper Berry: Protects against negativity. Clears and cleanses.
- ⤙ Vetiver: Protects.

Archangel Raguel — "Friend of God"

KEYWORD: Harmonious relationships

ASSOCIATIONS: Harmonious relationships, enthusiasm, kindness, wisdom, oversee archangels to work harmoniously together, justice, resolve arguments, group cooperation, defend the underdog, honor feelings, direction for loving and positive situations.

↞ Petitgrain: Promotes joy and harmony, especially in relationships. Promotes positive energy. Uplifts.

ADDITIONAL ESSENTIAL OILS:

↞ Rosemary: Inspires faith. Promotes enthusiasm.

↞ Orange: Uplifts. Promotes positive energy.

↞ Bergamot: Promotes self-love and positive energy. Opens heart to feeling.

Archangel Raphael — "God Heals"

KEYWORD: Healing

ASSOCIATIONS: Healing, healing on all levels, support and guidance for healers, heaven's physician, comfort, third eye, clairvoyance, stress relief, guidance for remedies via intuition.

BEST ESSENTIAL OIL:

↞ Lavender: Heals on all levels. Promotes acceptance. Eases stress and anxiety.

ADDITIONAL ESSENTIAL OILS:

↞ Rose: Heals wounds of the heart. Comforts. Eases stress and anxiety.

↞ Frankincense: Heals and strengthens spiritual consciousness. Comforts. Promotes slow and deep breathing. Eases stress and anxiety.

↞ Bay Laurel: Increases intuition.

+~ Palmarosa: Supports healing on all levels.
Promotes self-acceptance.

Archangel Raziel — "Secrets of God"

KEYWORD: Esoteric information

ASSOCIATIONS: Esoteric information, divine guidance, wizard of the angels, wisdom, kindness, intelligence, secrets of the universe, psychic abilities, manifesting, alchemist of the angels.

BEST ESSENTIAL OIL:

+~ Frankincense: Promotes spiritual wisdom and consciousness. Connects us to the eternal and the Divine.

ADDITIONAL ESSENTIAL OILS:

+~ Cedarwood: Strengthens the connection with the Divine. Promotes wisdom.

+~ Neroli: Promotes direct communication with guidance. Helps the manifestation of deepest and highest aspirations.

+~ Rosemary: Strengthens purpose and intent. Supports manifestation.

+~ Bay Laurel: Heightens intuitive abilities, especially clairaudience and clairvoyance.

+~ German Chamomile: Increases receptivity to intuitive messages.

+~ Myrrh: Supports earthly manifestations of dreams and visions.

Archangel Sandalphon — (meaning of name unclear)

KEYWORD: Prayers to God

ASSOCIATIONS: Carries prayers to God, speaking truth, peace, ability to receive, gentle yet powerful energy, twin to Metatron, one of only two archangels who were once mortal men, appreciation.

BEST ESSENTIAL OIL:

- ⤙ Myrrh: Bridges upper and lower energy centers, and heaven and earth. Promotes emotional harmony and peace.

ADDITIONAL ESSENTIAL OILS:

- ⤙ German Chamomile: Supports communication and speaking the truth. Calms. Promotes a sense of peace and gentleness. Increases ability to receive.

- ⤙ Jasmine: Promotes feelings of appreciation and gratitude.

- ⤙ Rose: Increases ability to receive. Helps release fear. Promotes a sense of peace.

- ⤙ Vetiver: Promotes feeling safe and secure.

Archangel Uriel — "The Light of God"

KEYWORD: Enlightenment

ASSOCIATIONS: Enlightenment, wisdom, inspiration, action, illuminate situations, subtle energy, clarity, prophetic information, one of the wisest archangels, speaking truth, support life purpose, integrity.

BEST ESSENTIAL OIL:

⤙ Lemon: Brings light into darkness. Promotes clarity, awareness, and inspiration. Energizes to take action.

ADDITIONAL ESSENTIAL OILS:

⤙ Frankincense: Strengthens spiritual consciousness. Promotes inspiration and wisdom.

⤙ German Chamomile: Promotes speaking the truth and receptivity to guidance.

⤙ Rosemary: Motivates to action. Promotes mental clarity.

⤙ Cypress: Promotes wisdom.

Archangel Zadkiel — "The Righteousness of God"

KEYWORD: Compassion

ASSOCIATIONS: Compassion, love, forgiveness, mercy, benevolence, faith, nonjudgment, patience, kindness.

BEST ESSENTIAL OIL:

⤙ Rose: Promotes compassion, love, and forgiveness.

ADDITIONAL ESSENTIAL OILS:

⤙ German Chamomile: Promotes forgiveness, patience, and kindness.

- Bergamot: Promotes positive energy, benevolence, and joy.
- Rosemary: Strengthens faith. Improves memory.
- Grapefruit: Clears and cleanses. Releases negative-emotion energy blocks.
- Bay Laurel: Opens us to new thoughts and perspectives.
- Cardamom: Encourages teaching others.

Key Angelic Essential Oils

- Basil: Helps to clear the mind to receive angelic guidance.
- Cedarwood: Helps to bring in the wisdom of the angels.
- German Chamomile: Helps to bring in the patience of the angels.
- Clary Sage: Helps to strengthen clairvoyance to connect with the angelic realm.
- Frankincense: Helps to bring in the secrets of the angels.
- Ginger: Helps to bring in the courage of the angels.

- Jasmine: The aroma favored by angels. Helps to bring you closer to angels and to bring in the beauty of the angels.
- Lavender: Helps to bring in the healing of the angels.
- Lemon: Helps to clear the mind for prophetic information from the angels.
- Myrrh: Helps to bring in the comfort of angels.
- Neroli: Helps to bring in the peace of the angels.
- Orange: Helps to bring in the joy of the angels.
- Petitgrain: Helps to bring in the justice of the angels.
- Pine: Helps to bring in the angels of nature.
- Rose: The aroma of angels. Helps to bring in the love and compassion of the angels.
- Rosemary: Helps to bring in the strength of the angels.
- Sandalwood: Helps to bring in the comfort of the angels.
- Thyme: Helps to bring in the protection of the angels.

Appendix V

Essential Oils
and Animal Associations

Just as essential oils have subtle and energetic qualities, as explored in this book, so too do animals. Traditional peoples, such as the Native American Cherokee and the ancient Chinese, have observed animals and consider certain ones to have these special qualities. The qualities are referred to as the animal's "power" or "medicine," which is identified by the animal's unique characteristics in the animal kingdom, such as being assertive or particularly intelligent.

Human personality traits can be associated with animals' medicine. If a person has mouse medicine, they have the ability to look closely and discern details. If they have eagle medicine, they can see the big picture from a high vantage point. In some traditional cultures, if you see or dream about a particular animal, you are to study that animal and its powers because its appearance is telling you to develop that quality in your life.

In this list, we identify animals whose medicine is associated with the essential oils presented in this book. If you would like to expand your scope of understanding of a particular essential oil, study the subtle properties of the animal associated with it. Our favorite reference books are *Animal-*

Speak (1996) and *Animal-Wise* (1999), both by Ted Andrews, and *Medicine Cards* (1988) by Jamie Sams and David Carson.

Spring is the season of the soul that signals optimism and hope. It is a time to clear away and release what no longer serves you—physically, mentally, emotionally, and spiritually—so that you can experience rebirth, inspiration, and renewed creativity. It is a time for new beginnings, new experiences, new relationships, and new perspectives on existing relationships. Spring is the season that represents the feminine, and also the childhood stage of your life.

- *Lemongrass*/Vulture (clears and cleanses): Vulture cleanses and clears away all that is "dead" or negative and sends it back to the earth.

- *Bay St. Thomas*/Hawk (releases fear): Hawk's fierce clear-sightedness pierces through fear and the confusion caused by fear.

- *Grapefruit*/Woodpecker (releases negative emotions): Woodpecker has great emotional strength, physical courage, and generosity of spirit that follow its own rhythm to release and overcome negative emotions.

- *Juniper Berry*/Cougar (protects against negativity and negative influences): Cougar, a silent hunter, has strength and craftiness and can avoid danger to successfully pursue its goals.

- *Orange*/Hummingbird (promotes joy): Hummingbird is a harbinger of joy, delight, and beauty.

- *Mandarin*/Dolphin (promotes optimism): Dolphin is playful, happy, and creative with an abundant belief in the promise of all good things.

- *Petitgrain*/Horse (promotes harmonious relationships): Horse has great power and intelligence that sensitively align and harmonize with others.

- *Bergamot*/Penguin (promotes hope): Penguin is loving, loyal, and ever-hopeful. It trusts and is trustworthy.

- *Geranium*/Swan (supports the feminine): Swan is exquisitely feminine, beautiful, graceful, and intuitive.

- *Coriander*/Beaver (promotes creativity): Beaver is the master builder of marvelous and intricate creations.

- *Nutmeg*/Crow (supports new beginnings): Crow is the master of magic who invokes new light from the cauldron of darkness.

⤙ *Eucalyptus*/Condor (promotes inspiration): Condor is inspiring as the largest of all flying birds with extraordinary vision and powerful flight. It is also known as the "sacred southern eagle."

Summer is the season of the soul that signals manifestation and full expression—the foundation for which is mental clarity, concentration, and focus. Your body, mind, heart, and spirit are energized and motivated, moving your thoughts into action. Fortitude, courage, and confidence help to bring your heart and soul's desire to fruition. Summer is the season that symbolizes the masculine and represents the young-adult stage of your life.

⤙ *Rosemary*/Kestrel (promotes mental clarity): Kestrel, a small falcon, has clear, focused attention and acute observational skills.

⤙ *Basil*/Panther (promotes concentration): Panther has the capacity to quietly and steadfastly concentrate and focus.

⤙ *Lemon*/Giraffe (promotes objectivity): Giraffe has the capacity to observe from a "higher" perspective.

- *Peppermint*/Bee (promotes mental energy): Bee has extraordinary energy and coordinated faculties.
- *Pine*/Moose (promotes willpower): Moose is powerful and dignified and has a strong will.
- *Cinnamon*/Raven (promotes confidence): Raven has a natural, easy, and humorous self-confidence.
- *Thyme*/Lion (supports the masculine): Lion has potent, male energy, power, and grace.
- *Tea Tree*/Otter (energizes on all levels): Otter is the embodiment of energy—physical and mental.
- *Clove*/Fox (motivates): Fox has a canny intelligence and the ability to motivate self and others.
- *Ginger*/Lynx (promotes manifesting): Lynx has a magical and mysterious ability to focus and manifest.
- *Ylang Ylang*/Porpoise (promotes passion and enthusiasm): Porpoise is creatively passionate and enthusiastic.
- *Fennel*/Salmon (promotes perseverance): Salmon has extraordinary strength of purpose and capacity to persevere against all odds.

DAILY AROMATHERAPY

Autumn is the season of the soul that signals a time to reflect on your life and assess the health and well-being of your body, mind, heart, and spirit. It is a time for insights and using good judgment regarding your relationships, how you take care of yourself, how you spend your time, and what you have accomplished. Forgiving and accepting your shortcomings, as well as the shortcomings of others, help you pave the way to a peaceful heart. It is also a time to acknowledge and be grateful for the many blessings in your life, and to be generous of spirit. In all of this, healing takes place. Autumn represents the mid-life stage of your life.

- *Spruce*/Wolf (supports self-reflection): Wolf has the ability to perceive, track, respond, and communicate, from a self-reflective place.
- *Fir*/Seal (supports self-understanding): Seal moves through water and air, emotions and mind, to understand the depths of the self.
- *Bay Laurel*/Elephant (promotes good judgment): Elephant has a powerful capacity to perceive and discern both the revealed and the hidden.
- *Clary Sage*/Snake (promotes intuition): Snake has a profound, grounded, intuitive knowing.

- *Palmarosa*/Dragonfly (promotes self-acceptance): Dragonfly heals the heart and mind in a way that is necessary to develop and strengthen self-acceptance.

- *Roman Chamomile*/Canary (supports forgiveness): Canary has the capacity to forgive self and others, opening the heart to allow a true song to come forth.

- *Marjoram*/Gazelle (helps to heal grief): Gazelle is graceful, lighthearted, emotionally mature, and able to gently process and release grief.

- *Lavender*/Bear (heals on all levels): Bear has the ability to navigate the different stages on the path of healing in a balanced way.

- *Jasmine*/Ladybug (promotes gratitude): Ladybug has a grateful appreciation for all of life's beauty, and the expected and unexpected ways in which hopes and dreams are fulfilled.

- *Cardamom*/Turkey (promotes generosity): Turkey is unconditionally generous, without thought or fear.

- *Cypress*/Coyote (supports personal growth): Coyote has the playful ability to engage in all experiences and use them as opportunities to grow. He is the "wise fool"—always growing and learning.

‑‑ *Rose*/Dove (promotes unconditional love):
Dove offers unconditional love and is gentle,
respectful, and peaceful.

Winter is the season of the soul that signals rest. It is a time
to feel comfortable, safe, and secure—in body, mind, heart,
and spirit. A sense of being *home* embraces you. There is an
awareness of wholeness, satisfaction, and abundance. It is a
time of peace and trust, and in that, there is restoration and
rejuvenation. It is a time when increasing wisdom can lead
the way to contemplative spirituality. Winter is the season
that represents the senior stage of your life.

‑‑ *Benzoin*/Dog (comfort): Dog has the
willingness to give and receive physical,
emotional, and spiritual comfort.

‑‑ *Vetiver*/Porcupine (feeling safe): Porcupine is
strong, well-protected, stable, and grounded,
with a consciousness of safety.

‑‑ *Vanilla*/Turtle (promotes feeling connected to
Mother Earth): Turtle embodies earth's
mothering, nurturing, and sustaining
qualities.

‑‑ *Oakmoss*/Buffalo (abundance): Buffalo has
the ability to gratefully receive and offer
abundant blessings on all levels—physical,
mental, emotional, and spiritual.

↠ *Neroli*/Goldfish (promotes a sense of peace): Goldfish has a peaceful, quiet, deep, and gentle nature.

↠ *Spikenard*/Cricket (promotes trust): Cricket has a basic trust in all things, especially the goodness of the universe.

↠ *Myrrh*/Deer (promotes the understanding of the spiritual perspective of emotional challenges): Deer has the ability and willingness to walk the spirit path into and through dark times with grace, purpose, and understanding.

↠ *Rosewood*/Whale (promotes spiritual opening and growth): Whale has a spiritual nature that is ever deepening, growing, expanding, and opening into new dimensions of wisdom.

↠ *Cedarwood*/Eagle (promotes a direct connection with the Divine): Eagle is intuitive and has a direct understanding of the holy, and offers an immediate connection with the Divine from both distant and close perspectives.

↠ *Sandalwood*/Cat (promotes a sense of oneness): Cat is wise, playful, and full of grace. It integrates body, mind, and spirit to achieve a sense of oneness with the self and the Divine.

⤙ *Elemi*/Butterfly (balances spiritual and worldly life): Butterfly has the ability to transform and integrate spirit and matter, body and soul.

⤙ *Frankincense*/Owl (encourages and supports spiritual wisdom): Owl has the ability to see into the darkness with enlightened wisdom.

Appendix VI
Subtle Anatomy

The subtle or energetic anatomy of your body is made up of *energy centers* and *subtle bodies.* There are seven primary energy centers, also known as chakras, located along the spine from the tailbone to the top of your head. They receive, assimilate, and transmit various forms of energy, playing an essential role in your state of consciousness and emotions.

The subtle bodies are levels that provide energy for the seven energy centers. These levels pass through the physical body outward from the skin. Though there are different interpretations, these levels are commonly identified as etheric (closest to the body), astral, mental, and spiritual (farthest from the body). Together they form an energetic structure that is referred to as your electromagnetic field, auric field, or energy field.

Essential oils can be used to affect your subtle anatomy. Many essential oils vibrate in harmony with the energy centers and can help keep them in balance. For more information on working with your subtle anatomy with essential oils, we recommend *Aromatherapy & Subtle Energy Techniques* (2000), our first book.

❧ The Energy Centers ❦

First Center — "Base Center"

COLOR: Red.

LOCATION: Base of the spine.

PHYSICAL ASSOCIATIONS: Intestines and adrenal glands.

MAIN CONCERNS: Self-preservation and survival.

ATTENDS TO: A strong, nurturing connection with Mother Earth, a sense of being grounded and stable, feeling secure and safe (lack of fear), feeling positive about life, a sense of abundance, health, vitality, feeling "at home" in the body and on the earth.

TEACHES: The embodiment of Spirit, and the sacredness of the physical world.

SUGGESTED ESSENTIAL OILS:

❧ Sandalwood, Vetiver, Oakmoss

Second Center — "Sacral Center"

COLOR: Orange.

LOCATION: Two inches below the navel.

PHYSICAL ASSOCIATIONS: The reproductive organs and glands.

MAIN CONCERNS: Relationships, creativity, creation, and sexuality.

ATTENDS TO: Allowing feelings to flow and be expressed, accessing enthusiasm about life, experiencing sensuality and pleasure, being creative, promoting positive personal growth and starting anew, encouraging or improving relationships, nurturing the feminine, experiencing emotional attachments.

TEACHES: The alignment of emotions and feelings with Spirit.

SUGGESTED ESSENTIAL OILS:

-+- Cardamom, Jasmine, Geranium, Ylang Ylang

Third Center — "Solar Plexus Center"

COLOR: Yellow.

LOCATION: Two inches above the navel.

PHYSICAL ASSOCIATIONS: Digestive system, liver, and pancreas.

MAIN CONCERNS: Personal power and will, self-worth, social identity, and likes and dislikes.

ATTENDS TO: Building confidence, self-acceptance, and self-esteem, assisting in achieving goals and manifesting, being responsible, developing personal will and integrity, accepting oneself, having self-worth, attracting what is wanted in life, being active, personal belief system, being confident, having energy, having courage, making choices, coping with change, protection from negativity.

TEACHES: Developing of personality in service to the Divine.

SUGGESTED ESSENTIAL OILS:

-+- Juniper Berry, Pine, Rosemary, Thyme

Fourth Center — "Heart Center"

COLOR: Green or pink.

LOCATION: Center of the chest.

PHYSICAL ASSOCIATIONS: Heart, lungs, and thymus gland.

MAIN CONCERNS: Love, compassion, the connection between friends and family.

ATTENDS TO: Nurturing oneself and others, unconditional love, connecting with community, discovering life's purpose, feeling and expressing compassion, joy, hope, devotion, gratitude, and peace, appreciating art and beauty, being empathetic, being emotionally warm and sincere, emotional attachments, meaningful relationships, being sympathetic, being generous, being patient.

TEACHES: The connection with the infinite, abundant love that is Spirit. Paying attention to the heart energy center will assist all the other centers.

SUGGESTED ESSENTIAL OILS:

⤜ Rose, Lavender, Bergamot, Mimosa

Fifth Center — "Throat Center"

COLOR: Sky blue.

LOCATION: Center of the throat.

PHYSICAL ASSOCIATIONS: Neck, throat, and thyroid gland.

MAIN CONCERNS: Communication (both speaking and listening).

ATTENDS TO: Expressing the truth freely, creative expression, being comfortable with silence, being able to listen to others as well as to one's inner voice, managing time well, connecting with divine will, self-expression, resolving inner conflicts, integrating new beliefs.

TEACHES: Personal will aligning with divine will to become an instrument of the sacred.

SUGGESTED ESSENTIAL OILS:

⤛ Roman Chamomile, German Chamomile, Geranium, Rosewood

Sixth Center — "Third Eye or Brow Center"

COLOR: Indigo or purple.

LOCATION: Forehead, just above and between the eyes.

PHYSICAL ASSOCIATIONS: Eyes, pituitary, and hypothalamus.

MAIN CONCERNS: Intellect, understanding, intuition, and dreams.

ATTENDS TO: Developing and balancing the intuitive and rational minds, assisting in memory and psychic development, self-reflection, increasing self-awareness and self-knowledge, dreams, imagination, intelligence, understanding, mental clarity, wisdom, good judgment, discernment, teaching others.

TEACHES: Healing, balancing, and expanding the human mind so it can be touched by the mind of Spirit.

SUGGESTED ESSENTIAL OILS:

⤛ Clary Sage, Bay Laurel, Fir, Basil

Seventh Center — "Crown Center"

COLOR: Violet or white.

LOCATION: Top of the head.

PHYSICAL ASSOCIATIONS: Brain, central nervous system, and pineal gland.

MAIN CONCERNS: Spirituality, faith, higher states of consciousness, enlightenment.

ATTENDS TO: Promoting spiritual growth, spiritual consciousness, and enlightenment, deepening faith, connecting with the Divine, sense of oneness, oneness of inner and outer life, aligning actions with the Divine, devotion to the Divine.

TEACHES: Surrendering to the mystery of the Divine, becoming one with Spirit.

SUGGESTED ESSENTIAL OILS:

⤙ Frankincense, Sandalwood, Cedarwood, Neroli

⤞ The Subtle Bodies ⤝

The *etheric body* lies directly outside of your physical body. It has a direct correlation with the state of your physical body and all of its sensations. It sustains the equilibrium between your physical body and your other subtle bodies, and houses an exact energetic replica of your physical body, providing a blueprint. This level is strengthened by good health, including physical exercise.

The *astral body* houses your feelings and emotions, and your relationships with people, animals, plants, your environment, and the universe. It affects your physical body through the nervous, endocrine, muscular, and immune systems. Positive emotions (love, joy, hope) expand the field while negative emotions (fear, anger, hatred) contract it. This level is strong when feelings, both negative and positive, are allowed to flow (not repressed), and when you have good relationships with people, giving importance to family, friends, and community.

The *mental body* houses intellectual function, rational thoughts, beliefs, judgments, the conscious and unconscious mind, and memories. This level is strengthened by activities such as learning, studying, and meditating.

The *spiritual body* houses your spiritual essence, and the knowing of your life's purpose. It connects you to your spiritual self and emotional experiences of divine love, spiritual joy, and bliss. Your spiritual body organizes the subtle bodies and holds them in association with the physical body. It provides a protective boundary where your energy ends and the rest of the world begins. This level is strengthened by maintaining harmony in your life, seeking higher truths, feeling connected to a greater purpose, and knowing you are a part of a divine plan.

Appendix VII
Essential Oil Safety

Because essential oils are concentrated, active plant extracts, care and responsibility must be taken with their use. Following are standard, recommended safety guidelines for using essential oils.

In *Daily Aromatherapy,* the aromas of the essential oils are inhaled through the nose. They are not applied to the skin.

1. Essential oils are for external use. Do not take essential oils internally.

2. Keep essential oils tightly closed and away from children.

3. Keep essential oils away from and out of your eyes. (If contact with eyes should occur, first put a drop of carrier oil such as canola, sweet almond, or sunflower oil in your eye to collect the essential oil, then flush well with water. If no carrier oil is available, try whole milk. If neither is available, flush profusely with water.)

4. Essential oils should be diluted before they are applied to the skin. (Standard dilution is 2%, which is 2 drops in 1 teaspoon of carrier, such as jojoba oil or fragrance-free lotion.)

5. If your skin becomes irritated with essential oils, rub the area with a carrier oil, and discontinue use.

6. Citrus oils extracted from the rinds can cause photosensitivity—discoloration and/or irritation of the skin when exposed to direct sunlight. It is recommended to avoid using citrus oils on your skin when exposed to the sun.

7. If you are allergy prone, test the essential oil under a bandage for twelve hours. If there is no reaction, the oil should be safe for you to use. If there is swelling or irritation, do not use the oil.

8. If you are pregnant, there are considerations for using essential oils. Refer to an essential oil specialist or an aromatherapy book that addresses this topic.

9. If you have a heart condition, there are considerations for using essential oils. Refer to an aromatherapy book that discusses this topic.

10. If you have any serious health problems, consult your physician before using essential oils.

11. If you are taking a homeopathic remedy, essential oils (most commonly Eucalyptus, Peppermint, and Rosemary) may negate its effect.

12. Essential oils are flammable. Do not use them near an open flame.

13. If you have epilepsy, do not use essential oils without consulting your physician.

14. If you have asthma, do not inhale essential oils without medical direction.

Appendix VIII
Aromatherapy 101

This book, *Daily Aromatherapy,* explores the psychological and subtle realms of essential oils to promote a sense of well-being. However, aromatherapy is also used for physical situations such as colds, muscle strain, and headaches. For those readers who are interested in learning about the broader scope of using aromatherapy for self-care, the following information, as well as suggested reading, is provided.

Introduction to Aromatherapy

Aromatherapy is the art and science of using the therapeutic properties of aromatic plant extracts known as essential oils to promote all levels of health and well-being—physical, psychological, and spiritual. It is an evolving modality that is valued for its effectiveness and wholistic nature in a variety of situations for natural self-care. It has been embraced by laypeople as well as professionals, including nurses, psychologists, aestheticians, and massage therapists.

Physically, essential oils have a range of properties that can relieve pain, soothe irritations, reduce inflammation, relax muscles, support the immune system, promote wound healing, stimulate circulation, fight a broad spectrum of infections (bacteria, fungi, viruses), and beautify the complexion.

This is achieved primarily by the chemical constituents of which essential oils are composed. For example, *oxides* have expectorant qualities, making them useful for respiratory congestion. *Aldehydes* reduce inflammation and are calming. *Esters* balance and soothe. However, the synergy of the chemical constituents in an essential oil sometimes produces results that cannot be explained by chemical evaluation or scientific means. For this reason, empirical evidence and experience are a valued and respected part of the body of aromatherapy knowledge and information.

Psychologically, aromatherapy is used to promote positive or desired mental and emotional states such as clarity, concentration, joy, and optimism, and to reduce negative mental or emotional states such as lack of focus, mental fatigue, depression, anxiety, anger, and fear. This is achieved primarily in three ways: 1) by using an essential oil with the desired physical effects, such as Roman Chamomile, which sedates the nervous system, to help mentally relax and relieve stress, 2) by smelling a favorite essential oil that is simply pleasurable and uplifts your mood, and 3) by using memory and association with an aroma to create and re-create positive feelings. In the latter case, a pleasant-smelling essential oil is used in conjunction with a pleasant experience. When repeated, the pleasant experience and the scent lock together in your memory. When this occurs, simply smelling the essential oil can re-create the positive feelings associated with the pleasant experience. This technique is often used successfully with guided imagery.

Spiritually, aromatherapy is used to assist transformation techniques such as meditation, affirmation, visualization, and prayer. Aromas have been used for hundreds of years for this purpose. The spiritual use of essential oils is often referred to as *subtle aromatherapy* and is based on the subtle energy system of your body, as described in Appendix VI. When used in this way, the essential oil is chosen for its energetic or vibrational properties. (See *Vibrational Medicine* (2001) by Richard Gerber.) Different essential oils have different energetic qualities. These are determined by 1) the traditional uses of the essential oil and possibly the herb of the same plant, 2) the physical and psychological effects of the essential oil, 3) the gesture and the signature of the plant itself (its appearance and characteristics), and 4) personal experience.

When you use essential oils, their effects cannot be completely separated or isolated into one realm or the other of body, mind, or spirit. For example, when you use Lavender to soothe sunburn, the aroma will also have a soothing effect on the mind. This demonstrates the true wholistic nature of essential oils, which aligns so beautifully with the wholistic nature of human beings.

Aromatherapy, as an alternative or complementary therapeutic modality, requires using genuine and authentic essential oils. Such oils are pure and unadulterated and have been extracted from vital plants that have been properly grown, harvested, and distilled. (Synthetic fragrances are not used in aromatherapy.) It is interesting to note that essential oils' unique compositions and therapeutic properties cannot be synthetically duplicated in a laboratory.

The History of Aromatherapy

R. M. Gattefossé, a French chemist and perfumer, is considered the father of modern aromatherapy. In the early 1920s, Gattefossé seriously burned his hand in his laboratory and immersed it in the only liquid close and available, a vat of Lavender oil. To his amazement, the burn lost its redness and the pain diminished rapidly. As days passed, it healed much sooner than he expected. He was so impressed with this reaction that he began investigating the medicinal properties of essential oils and dedicated the rest of his life to this research, coining the term "aromatherapy" in 1928.

There was not much initial interest in Gattefossé's work and when World War II broke out, interest in aromatherapy all but disappeared. It was not until 1964 that real interest began. At this time, Dr. Jean Valnet, a French medical doctor, was inspired by Gattefossé's research and published *Aromatherapie: The Treatment of Illness with the Essence of Plants.* Dr. Valnet went on to use essential oils (those with superior antiseptic qualities) to treat wounds and infections, to fumigate hospital wards, and to sterilize surgical instruments. Two of Valnet's students, Margarite Maury and Micheline Arcier, brought aromatherapy to England and used it for massage and skin care. Madame Maury later became respected for her research on both the physical and psychological effects of essential oils.

In 1977, Robert Tisserand discovered Valnet's book on a visit to France from his native England. He translated it and published *The Art of Aromatherapy* in 1979, bringing the book to the English-speaking world. In the mid-1980s, aromatherapy gained a foothold in the United States. The National Association for Holistic Aromatherapy emerged in the early 1990s as a fellowship of professionals and laypeople who advocated aromatherapy as a self-help modality. Today, there is continued interest and research to substantiate aromatherapy's effectiveness and range of applications. Aromatherapy is recognized in complementary and alternative medicine (CAM) and is being used in the fields of medicine, psychology, wholistic health, massage therapy, cosmetology, and energy healing.

The Nature of Essential Oils

Essential oils are highly concentrated—one hundred times stronger than the dried herb of the same plant. They exist in a variety of colors and viscosities. For example, Bergamot is green and watery whereas Benzoin is amber and thick. Essential oils are soluble in alcohol and vegetable oils. They are not soluble in water. They will last for many years when properly stored in dark glass bottles with tight fitting caps away from heat and light. Essential oils do not become rancid because they do not contain fatty acids. Different essential oils have different volatility rates. Many will evaporate quickly into the air if left in an open container. Others evaporate slowly.

The quality and therapeutic properties of a specific essential oil depend on the soil in which the plant is grown, the climate, location, amount of sun exposure, amount of water received, time of extraction, and method of distillation. Some plants produce an abundance of essential oils whereas others produce very little. The concentration of essential oil in the plant and how it is extracted will dictate its price. For example, Peppermint and Eucalyptus produce large amounts of essential oil and are relatively inexpensive. Rose produces very little, taking up to three thousand pounds of petals to produce one pound of essential oil. As a result, it is one of the most expensive and prized essential oils.

Various plant parts are used to produce different essential oils. As examples, flowers are used for Rose, leaves for Eucalyptus, roots for Vetiver, fruit seeds for Coriander, wood for Sandalwood, bark for Cinnamon, resin for Myrrh, and rind for citrus oils such as Orange, Lemon, and Lime. (**Note:** The oils produced from citrus rind are more accurately called *essences.* By definition, they are not true essential oils.)

An essential oil must be carefully extracted at the right stage of plant development, using the right method of extraction, in order to preserve the oil's valuable therapeutic properties. The method of extraction must suit the plant while protecting the essential oil. The most common is distillation—water distillation, water and steam distillation, or steam distillation. Cold expression extraction (the use of pressure) is primarily used for citrus oils. Other methods include the use of solvents to produce an *absolute,* and carbon dioxide to produce a CO_2 extraction. Research and experimentation continue to look for new and more effective methods of extraction to obtain an essential oil, while preserving its natural and complete properties.

How Essential Oils Affect Us

Essential oils are used to promote health and well-being by application to the skin and by inhalation (aromatic molecules entering the nose). The most common methods are via massage, bath, compress, steam inhalation, and diffusion. Because essential oils are so highly concentrated, they are diluted before use, whether it is for a physical, psychological, or subtle energy purpose. In the case of essential oils, more is not necessarily better.

When applied to the skin, essential oils' small molecular structure and attraction-to-oil *(lipophilic)* characteristics allow certain constituents to be absorbed into the skin, where they enter the bloodstream through small capillaries, circulate throughout the body, and are eliminated through the sweat glands and other body functions.

When the aroma of an essential oil is inhaled through the nose, some molecules enter the lungs and others contact the olfactory bulb. In the lungs, the odor molecules enter the bloodstream and circulate through the body, as described above. Those connecting with the olfactory bulb travel to the limbic part of the brain and produce or affect emotional responses, memories, instinctual drives, and glandular functions via the hypothalamus.

Suggested Reading

-+ *Aromatherapy: Soothing Remedies* (2002) by Valerie Gennari Cooksley, RN

-+ *Vibrational Medicine* (2001) by Richard Gerber, MD

-+ *Clinical Aromatherapy* (2003) by Jane Buckle

-+ *Advanced Aromatherapy* (1998) by Dr. Kurt Schnaubelt

About the Authors

Joni Keim has been working in the alternative health field since 1976 as an educator,
author, practitioner, and consultant. She
has certificates in aromatherapy, holistic
health sciences, massage, aesthetics, flower
essence therapy, and energy healing. Keim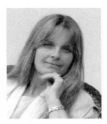
is a technical advisor and educator for the Natural Product
Industry and for the professional aromatherapy field. She has
a private consulting practice in Sonoma County specializing
in creating proprietary aromatherapy blends, designing for-
mulation guidelines for natural skin care products, and integrating alternative modalities into wellness and spa programs.

Ruah Bull, MA, MEd, has been working
in the healing arts since 1978. She holds
master's degrees in education and psychology, and certificates in spiritual direction, guided imagery, aromatherapy, and
energy healing. Bull has a private practice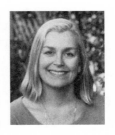
in spiritual direction working with people on both traditional
and non-traditional spiritual paths. She lives in Sonoma
County, California.